GENTAMICIN

BIOSYNTHESIS, MEDICINAL APPLICATIONS AND POTENTIAL SIDE EFFECTS

PHARMACOLOGY - RESEARCH, SAFETY TESTING AND REGULATION

Additional books in this series can be found on Nova's website under the Series tab.

Additional e-books in this series can be found on Nova's website under the e-book tab.

PHARMACOLOGY - RESEARCH, SAFETY TESTING AND REGULATION

GENTAMICIN

BIOSYNTHESIS, MEDICINAL APPLICATIONS AND POTENTIAL SIDE EFFECTS

EMILIE KRUGER
EDITOR

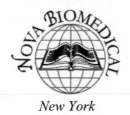

New York

For permission to use material from this book please contact us:
Telephone 631-231-7269; Fax 631-231-8175
Web Site: http://www.novapublishers.com

NOTICE TO THE READER

The Publisher has taken reasonable care in the preparation of this book, but makes no expressed or implied warranty of any kind and assumes no responsibility for any errors or omissions. No liability is assumed for incidental or consequential damages in connection with or arising out of information contained in this book. The Publisher shall not be liable for any special, consequential, or exemplary damages resulting, in whole or in part, from the readers' use of, or reliance upon, this material. Any parts of this book based on government reports are so indicated and copyright is claimed for those parts to the extent applicable to compilations of such works.

Independent verification should be sought for any data, advice or recommendations contained in this book. In addition, no responsibility is assumed by the publisher for any injury and/or damage to persons or property arising from any methods, products, instructions, ideas or otherwise contained in this publication.

This publication is designed to provide accurate and authoritative information with regard to the subject matter covered herein. It is sold with the clear understanding that the Publisher is not engaged in rendering legal or any other professional services. If legal or any other expert assistance is required, the services of a competent person should be sought. FROM A DECLARATION OF PARTICIPANTS JOINTLY ADOPTED BY A COMMITTEE OF THE AMERICAN BAR ASSOCIATION AND A COMMITTEE OF PUBLISHERS.

Additional color graphics may be available in the e-book version of this book.

Library of Congress Cataloging-in-Publication Data

ISBN: 978-1-62808-841-0

Library of Congress Control Number: 2013947023

Published by Nova Science Publishers, Inc. † New York

CONTENTS

Contents

PREFACE

Gentamicin is an aminoglycoside antibiotic naturally synthesized by Micromonospora, a Gram-positive genus of bacteria widely found in water and soil. This antibiotic is useful against a wide variety of bacteria, and works by binding the 30S subunit of the bacterial ribosome, which interrupts bacterial protein synthesis. In this book, the authors discuss the biosynthesis, medicinal applications and potential side effects of Gentamicin. Topics include Gentamicin used in combination therapy and applied to medicinal materials for clinical applications; use of natural products to enhance the antibiotic activity of Gentamicin and other aminoglycosides; regiospecific Gentamicin functionalization; Gentamicin and particle engineering; and the indications and adverse effects of Gentamicin.

Chapter 1 – Gentamicin (GM) was discovered in 1963 and was introduced into parenteral usage in 1971. Since then, GM has been widely used in medicinal applications. The Food and Drug Administration (FDA) of the United States approved the routine prescription of GM to treat the following infectious disorders: infection due to *Klebsiella pneumoniae, Escherichia coli, Serratia marcescens, Citrobacter* spp., *Enterobacteriaceae* spp., *Pseudomonas* spp.; *Staphylococcus* infectious disease; bacterial meningitis; bacterial sepsis of newborns; bacterial septicemia; infection of the eye, bone, skin and/or subcutaneous tissue; infective endocarditis; peritoneal dialysis–associated peritonitis due to *Pseudomonas* and other gram-negative organisms; peritonitis due to gastrointestinal tract infections; respiratory tract infections; and urinary tract infectious disease.

GM is an old antibiotic and is used widely beyond its FDA-labeled indications as follows: actinomycotic infection; *Staph. saprophyticus* bacteremia with pyelonephritis; appendicitis; cystic fibrosis; diverticulitis;

adjunct regimen for febrile neutropenia; female genital infection; uterine infection; postnatal infection; necrotizing enterocolitis in fetus or newborn; osteomyelitis; pelvic inflammatory disease; plague; gonorrhea; tularemia; prophylaxis of post-cholecystectomy infection, transrectal prostate biopsy, and post–tympanostomy-related infection; malignant otitis externa; and intratympanically or transtympanically for Ménière's disease. GM is also used in combination regimens, such as with beta-lactam antibiotics to treat mixed infection and with bacteriophage to treat *Staph. aureus* infections. It is also added to medical materials, such as GM-loaded cement spacers for osteomyelitis and prosthetic joint–associated infections.

Overall, there are many medicinal applications for GM. To reduce the development of GM-resistant bacteria and to maintain its effectiveness, GM should be used only to treat or prevent infections that are proven or strongly suspected as being caused by susceptible bacteria. In the future, the authors believe that GM will be used more widely in combination therapy and applied to medical materials for clinical applications. A definitive, appropriately powered study of this antibiotic and its clinical applications is now required, especially in terms of its effectiveness, safety, and cost.

Chapter 2 – Gentamicin sulfate (GS) is one of the most important antibiotics of the family "Aminoglycosides" worldwide used for its effective bactericidal activities, low bacterial resistance and post-antibiotic effects, and moderate cost. GS, similarly to other members of the "aminoglycosides" family, shows low effectiveness when administered orally, therefore, the antibiotic is usually administered intravenously or intramuscularly. However, due to its pharmacokinetics and biopharmaceutical properties, multiple systemic daily administrations are needed to achieve good antibiotic concentrations; this may cause serious side effects such as ototoxicity and nephrotoxicity which limit its clinical exploitation.

A local administration which can deliver high dose of drug directly to the site of infection, while minimizing systemic exposure, can overcome these limits. In this case, appropriate dosage forms must be designed to obtain a local controlled drug release and to solve biopharmaceutical and pharmacokinetic issues that hinder the optimal use of GS in the clinical practice.

In the last few years microtechnologies have been applied as tool to innovate GS delivery. The major drawback encountered when formulating GS microparticles is its high hygroscopicity. In fact, as it is well known, hygroscopicity may modulate the moisture content of microparticles in the final dosage form and it is correlated to chemical or physical instability and poor flowability of the final powder product.

The present chapter briefly describes the critical properties of gentamicin from both a pharmacological and technological point of view.

Particularly, the aim of the chapter is to illustrates "particle engineering" strategies, i.e. spray drying and supercritical fluid techniques, adopted to improve technological properties of GS raw material. A special focus will be on i) the development of dry powders for inhalation, ii) the development of microparticulate powder for topical application in wound care. Both approaches allow to obtain micronized gentamicin powders, easy to handle, stable for long time and suitable for pulmonary and topical administration, respectively.

Chapter 3 – The capacity to develop resistance to antibacterial agents is a characteristic observed among microorganisms in general. Bacteria are able to develop different mechanisms of resistance, which are genetically coded, where resistance genes can be acquired through mutation and transfer of genetic material.

Essential oils consist of volatile elements, which are present in many plant organs, are related to various functions necessary for the survival of the plant, exerting a fundamental role in the defense against microorganisms and offering protection.

The use of extracts and essential oils of plants as antimicrobial agents shows a low possibility that microorganisms will acquire resistance to their action, because they are complex mixtures, making microbial adaptation very difficult.

The chapter discuss the activity of isolated substances isolated citronellol, citronellal and myrcene on bacterial resistance in combination with antibiotics using direct and gaseous contact methods.

Chapter 4 – Gentamicin is an aminoglycoside antibiotic naturally synthesized by *Micromonospora*, a Gram-positive genus of bacteria widely found in water and soil. This antibiotic is useful against a wide variety of bacteria, and works by binding the 30S subunit of the bacterial ribosome, which interrupts bacterial protein synthesis. High serum concentrations of gentamicin can result in permanent damage to the balance and orientation components of the inner ear, and can have nephrotoxic effects in renal cells, potentially leading to renal failure.

Gentamicin is a complex consisting of several structurally different components. The three major constituents the gentamicin complex, C1, C2, and C1a, differ only by the presence or absence of methyl groups in different locations on each molecule, the relative proportions of which can vary widely depending on how the antibiotic was cultured or isolated. Each component has five different amino groups and three hydroxyl groups, and contains two acid sensitive glycosidic linkages. The presence of these multiple reactive groups in each component present considerable challenges to selective modification of gentamicin.

It would thus be useful to be able to regiospecifically functionalize gentamicin in order to tailor the derivatization to meet the needs of a particular application. This paper will describe a variety of methods that have proven useful for the regiospecific functionalization of gentamicin at different locations.

Chapter 5 – Gentamicin is an antibiotic agent, belonging to the aminoglycosides group, which acts joining the ribosoma subunits 30S and 50S and blocking the translation of mRNA in the initial phase of protein synthesis, originating non-functional proteins in susceptible microorganisms. Its bactericidal activity is concentration-dependent and is slightly influenced by the bacterial inoculum amount; the duration of the antibiotic effect ranges between 0.5-7 hours, depending on the concentration of antibiotic and the exposure time to the drug.

Gentamicin acts inside the bacterial cell. This occurs in two stages by an active transport mechanism. In the first phase, the entrance into the cell depends on the transmembrane potential generated by aerobic metabolism. The second phase is favoured by the previous union of the aminoglycoside to the bacterial ribosome. Certain conditions that reduce the electrical potential of the membrane, such as anaerobic status or low pH of the medium, decrease the income of these compounds into the bacterial cytoplasm.

Once inside the cell, aminoglycosides join in an irreversible way the subunit 30S of the bacterial ribosome. This union interferes with the elongation of the peptide chain. They also cause incorrect translation of the genetic code, performing altered proteins. Some of these are membrane proteins and the result is the formation of channels that allow the entrance of more drug into the cell.

Specifically, gentamicin is active against gram-negative aerobic bacilli, including *Enterobacteriaceae* and non-fermenting microorganisms (excepting *Stenotrophomona maltophilia* and Burkholderia cepacia). It shows antibiotic action against Staphylococci (*S. aureus* and *S. epidermidis*), including penicillinase-producing strains, but presents limited activity against *Streptococci*, lacking any activity against anaerobic bacteria and *Mycobacteria*. It is the most effective aminoglycoside against *Serratia* and

Brucella, and presents the best synergic effect against *Streptococci, Enterococcus, Staphylococci* and *Listeria,* when combined with beta-lactam agents or vancomycin.

The cut-off point to determine the sensitivity of a microorganism to this antibiotic is with a CMI≤4 mg/L. On the other hand, a bacteria can be considered resistant to gentamicin when presenting a CMI≥16 mg/L. The maximal effect is obtained at concentrations of 6 - 10 mg/L with doses of 1.5 mg/kg iv or im. Gentamicin presents renal elimination at 90% and 10% with the bile.

In: Gentamicin
Editor: Emilie Kruger

ISBN: 978-1-62808-841-0
© 2013 Nova Science Publishers, Inc.

Chapter 1

MEDICINAL APPLICATION OF GENTAMICIN: FROM PAST TO FUTURE

Changhua Chen,[1,] Yumin Chen[2] and Baoyuan Chen[2]*

[1]Division of Infectious Diseases, Department of Internal
Medicine, Changhua Christian Hospital, Changhua, Taiwan
[2]Department of Pharmacy, Changhua Christian
Hospital, Changhua, Taiwan

ABSTRACT

Gentamicin (GM) was discovered in 1963 and was introduced into parenteral usage in 1971. Since then, GM has been widely used in medicinal applications. The Food and Drug Administration (FDA) of the United States approved the routine prescription of GM to treat the following infectious disorders: infection due to *Klebsiella pneumoniae, Escherichia coli, Serratia marcescens, Citrobacter* spp., *Enterobacteriaceae* spp., *Pseudomonas* spp.; *Staphylococcus* infectious disease; bacterial meningitis; bacterial sepsis of newborns; bacterial septicemia; infection of the eye, bone, skin and/or subcutaneous tissue; infective endocarditis; peritoneal dialysis–associated peritonitis due to *Pseudomonas* and other gram-negative organisms; peritonitis due to

---

* Corresponding author: Changhua Chen, Division of Infectious Diseases, Department of Internal Medicine, Changhua Christian Hospital, 135 Nanhsiau Street, Changhua, Taiwan. E-mail address: changhua@cch.org.tw.

gastrointestinal tract infections; respiratory tract infections; and urinary tract infectious disease.

GM is an old antibiotic and is used widely beyond its FDA-labeled indications as follows: actinomycotic infection; *Staph. saprophyticus* bacteremia with pyelonephritis; appendicitis; cystic fibrosis; diverticulitis; adjunct regimen for febrile neutropenia; female genital infection; uterine infection; postnatal infection; necrotizing enterocolitis in fetus or newborn; osteomyelitis; pelvic inflammatory disease; plague; gonorrhea; tularemia; prophylaxis of post-cholecystectomy infection, transrectal prostate biopsy, and post–tympanostomy-related infection; malignant otitis externa; and intratympanically or transtympanically for Ménière's disease. GM is also used in combination regimens, such as with beta-lactam antibiotics to treat mixed infection and with bacteriophage to treat *Staph. aureus* infections. It is also added to medical materials, such as GM-loaded cement spacers for osteomyelitis and prosthetic joint–associated infections.

Overall, there are many medicinal applications for GM. To reduce the development of GM-resistant bacteria and to maintain its effectiveness, GM should be used only to treat or prevent infections that are proven or strongly suspected as being caused by susceptible bacteria. In the future, we believe that GM will be used more widely in combination therapy and applied to medical materials for clinical applications. A definitive, appropriately powered study of this antibiotic and its clinical applications is now required, especially in terms of its effectiveness, safety, and cost.

ABBREVIATIONS

ALCS	Antibiotic-loaded cement spacer
AMP	Ampicillin
CABG	Coronary artery bypass graft
CDM	Clindamycin
CF	Cystic fibrosis
CL	Cutaneous leishmaniasis
CRKP	Carbapenem-resistant *Klebsiella pneumoniae*
CRS	Chronic rhinosinusitis
DOX	Doxycycline
EOS	Early-onset neonatal sepsis
ESI	Exit site infections
FDA	Food and Drug Administration
GM	Gentamicin

GN	Gram-negative
HS	Hidradenitis suppurativa
ITD	Intratympanic dexamethasone
ITG	Intratympanic gentamicin
IV	Intravenous
MD	Ménière's disease
MTD	Metronidazole
MIC	Minimum inhibitory concentration
NEC	Necrotizing enterocolitis
PC	Primary closure
PD	Peritoneal dialysis
PEN	Penicillin
PID	Pelvic inflammatory disease
PJI	Prosthetic joint infection
PREHAB	Prehabilitation
RCT	Randomized controlled trial
SDD	Selective digestive decontamination
SSI	Surgical site infection
SWI	Sternal wound infection
TA	Triamcinolone acetonide
TMP-SMX	Trimethoprim-sulfamethoxazole
uVD	Unilateral vestibular deafferentation
US	United States
VOR	Vestibulo-ocular reflex

INTRODUCTION

Gentamicin (GM) is an aminoglycoside that is widely used in clinical conditions to fair clinical response. It was isolated from *Micromonospora* in 1963, proving to be a breakthrough in the treatment of gram-negative (GN) bacillary infections, including those caused by *Pseudomonas aeruginosa*. It was introduced into parenteral usage in 1971. GM has been widely used in medicinal applications since then. In the past 50 years, the clinical outcome of GM use tended to be good, but the opposite was sometimes true. Due to the progression of pharmaceuticals, the prescription of GM has decreased.

Based on clinical experience where the response to GM is good, the United States (US) Food and Drug Administration (FDA) approved the use of GM for treating the following infectious disorders: infection by *Klebsiella pneumoniae, Escherichia coli, Serratia marcescens, Citrobacter* spp., *Enterobacteriaceae* spp., or *Pseudomonas* spp.; *Staphylococcus* infectious disease; bacterial meningitis; bacterial sepsis of newborns; bacterial septicemia; infection of the eye, bone, skin and/or subcutaneous tissue; infective endocarditis; peritoneal dialysis (PD)-associated peritonitis due to *Pseudomonas* and other GN organisms; peritonitis due to gastrointestinal tract infections; respiratory tract infection; and urinary tract infectious disease. GM is also used widely beyond its FDA-labeled indications as follows: actinomycotic infection; *Staph. saprophyticus* bacteremia with pyelonephritis; appendicitis; cystic fibrosis (CF); diverticulitis; adjunct regimen for febrile neutropenia; female genital infection; uterine infection; peripartum and postnatal infection; necrotizing enterocolitis (NEC) in fetus or newborn; osteomyelitis; pelvic inflammatory disease (PID); plague; gonorrhea; tularemia; prophylaxis of post-cholecystectomy infection, transrectal prostate biopsy, and post–tympanostomy-related infection; malignant otitis externa; and intratympanically or transtympanically for Ménière's disease (MD). GM is also used in combination regimens, such as with beta-lactam antibiotics to treat mixed infections and with bacteriophage to treat *Staph. aureus* infections. GM is also added to medical materials, such as GM-loaded cement spacers for osteomyelitis and prosthetic joint-associated infections (PJIs). The application of GM has changed in recent years.

This chapter aims to provide physicians and pharmacists with a review of GM and its role in the treatment of infectious diseases, with focus on its medicinal applications.

There is more than 50 years' worth of cumulative clinical experience behind GM; as less adverse reactions are reported, and it is cheap and convenient, GM continues to play an important role in the treatment and prophylaxis of infectious and non-infectious diseases even in the face of patient-centered treatment, quality of medical care in general, resistant microorganisms, cost–benefit limitations, and overall medical expenses.

CLINICAL APPLICATIONS

Section 1. Medicinal Application of GM in the Past

GM exerts concentration-dependent bactericidal action and is active against a wide range of aerobic GN bacilli. GM is also active against staphylococci and certain mycobacteria.

It is effective even when the bacterial inoculum is large, and resistance rarely develops during the course of treatment. Due to its potency, GM is used as prophylaxis and treatment in a variety of clinical situations.

Over the course of half a century, GM has been used in the treatment and prophylaxis of infectious and non-infectious diseases that constitute more than 40 clinical conditions. We have divided the use of GM into FDA-approved and non–FDA-approved labeling indications. These indications are summarized in Table 1, and are introduced in turn in the following sections.

Table 1. FDA-approved and non–FDA-approved labeling indications

	FDA-approved labeling indications	Non–FDA-approved labeling indications
Pathogen-related	Infection due to *Enterobacteriaceae*, *Escherichia coli*, *Klebsiella pneumoniae*, *Serratia marcescens*, *Pseudomonas* spp., *Citrobacter* spp., *Proteus* spp., *Staphylococcus* spp., peritoneal dialysis-associated peritonitis due to *Pseudomonas* and other gram-negative organisms	Infection due to *Actinomyces*, *Clostridium perfringens*, plague (caused by *Yersinia pestis*), and tularemia (caused by *Francisella tularensis*)
Disease-related	Bacterial meningitis, ocular infection, infective endocarditis, respiratory tract infection, peritonitis and other gastrointestinal tract infections, urinary tract infectious disease, infection of bone, skin, and/or subcutaneous tissue, bacterial septicemia	Appendicitis, cat scratch disease, diarrhea, diverticulitis, female genital infection, infection of uterus, peripartum and postnatal infection, malignant otitis externa, Ménière's disease, necrotizing enterocolitis in fetus or newborn, osteomyelitis, pelvic inflammatory disease, cystic fibrosis, decubitus ulcer
Prophylaxis		Prophylaxis of postoperative infection of the nervous system, eye surgery, tympanostomy, postoperative infection on head and neck-related surgery, bacterial endocarditis, neutropenic status, burns

A. FDA-Approved Labeling Indications

Numerous clinical reports for GM prescription were published in the 1970s. Its FDA-approved labeling indications included at least 18 clinical conditions. We have categorized the conditions according to whether they are pathogen or disease-oriented.

The pathogen-oriented conditions include infection due to *Enterobacteriaceae* spp., *E. coli, K. pneumoniae, Pseudomonas* spp., *Citrobacter* spp., *Proteus* spp., *S. marcescens*; PD-associated peritonitis due to *Pseudomonas* and other GN organisms; and Staphylococcus infectious disease. In 1996, Anon wrote that a third-generation cephalosporin was the preferred treatment of *K. pneumoniae* infections and that an aminoglycoside such as GM was an alternative choice and may be added to a third-generation cephalosporin in cases of severe illness; GM was also an alternative for treatment of indole-positive *Proteus* infections [1].

In studies from the 1970s, Levinsky described 2 patients with *Pseudomonas* osteomyelitis (1 infant and one 12-year-old) who responded satisfactorily to surgery and antibiotic therapy involving GM with carbenicillin over 6 weeks [2]. Madsen et al. and Walker and Gentry reported that GM was effective in complicated urinary tract infections due to *P. aeruginosa* [3, 4]. GM has been administered intraperitoneally for PD-associated peritonitis. It was also indicated for the treatment of serious infections caused by *P. aeruginosa* and other susceptible organisms [5].

Smolin reported a fair response to GM over 8 postoperative days in a patient with *Proteus* endophthalmitis following cataract surgery in the right eye [6]. And Kourtopoulos and Khan reported that GM was useful in *S. marcescens* meningitis and initially effective in *S. marcescens* endocarditis in a heroin addict [7, 8]. Its product information states that GM is approved for serious infections caused by *Citrobacter* spp., *Enterobacter* spp., and *E. coli*. GM is effective in the treatment of *Staphylococcus* spp. (coagulase-positive and coagulase-negative) infections.

For methicillin-resistant *Staph. aureus* or *Staph. epidermidis* infections, GM with or without both vancomycin and rifampin is recommended as the therapy of choice [1, 5].

Many clinical conditions for GM usage were reported in the 1970s. The disease-oriented conditions include bacterial meningitis, ocular infection, infective endocarditis, respiratory tract infection, peritonitis and other gastrointestinal tract infections, urinary tract infectious disease, infection of bone or skin with/without subcutaneous tissue, and bacterial septicemia.

Our literature review indicates that GM was recommended as adjunctive therapy for the treatment of bacterial meningitis caused by laboratory-isolated pathogens of *Listeria monocytogenes, Streptococcus agalactiae*, or *P. aeruginosa*, and combination treatment involving GM was recommended for the treatment of meningitis caused by *Enterococcus* spp. [9-12].

Many authors wrote that GM should be used in combination with other antibiotics. GM ophthalmic solution and ointment are effective for treating ocular bacterial infections caused by susceptible microorganisms. GM ophthalmic solution and ointment have been indicated in the topical treatment of a variety of ocular infections [13-14].

GM in combination with appropriate antimicrobial therapy (penicillins, cephalosporins, or vancomycin) was recommended for the treatment of streptococcal, staphylococcal, enterococcal, and culture-negative (including *Bartonella*) endocarditis [5, 15-16], but was not proven to decrease mortality. GM is effective in respiratory infections caused by susceptible GN bacilli.

Sharma reported that once-daily administration of GM for 7–10 days was associated with complete clinical resolution of signs and symptoms in 93% of patients with uncomplicated, acute, recurrent, or chronic urinary tract infections [17].

GM was effective in the treatment of complicated urinary tract infection caused by GN bacilli [18]. Topical 0.1% GM sulfate cream and ointment is indicated for primary skin infections, including impetigo contagiosa, superficial folliculitis, ecthyma, furunculosis, sycosis barbae, and pyoderma gangrenosum, and for secondary skin infections such as infectious eczematoid dermatitis, pustular acne, pustular psoriasis, infected seborrheic dermatitis, infected contact dermatitis (including poison ivy), infected excoriations, and bacterial superinfections of fungal or viral infections [5, 19-21].

The studies of the 1970s reported that GM was effective in the treatment of septicemia caused by susceptible GN bacilli in adults and children. Concomitant use of an antipseudomonal penicillin (PEN) is indicated in *Pseudomonas* bacteremia. GM has also been proven effective in *S. marcescens* septicemia and septicemia due to *Yersinia* enterocolitica.

Its use in the treatment of septicemia caused by susceptible GN bacilli in adults and children is also effective [22-26]. According to its product information, GM is approved for serious bone infections and serious gastrointestinal tract infections caused by susceptible bacteria [5].

In 1980–1990, the clinical experience of GM was one of fair response and low medical expense.

B. Non–FDA-Approved Labeling Indications

The clinical presentations of diseases can be varied and complicated. Due to poor clinical response to traditional treatment, the availability of preliminary results only (e.g., results of clinical experience or from animal studies but not approved by FDA), and low cost, GM has been used in non–FDA-approved labeling indications. The non–FDA-approved labeling indications include at least 27 clinical conditions. We have categorized these conditions as pathogen-oriented conditions, disease treatment conditions, and disease prophylaxis conditions.

The pathogen-oriented conditions include actinomycotic infection, bacterial septicemia, e.g., infection due to *Clostridium perfringens*, plague (caused by *Y. pestis*), and tularemia (caused by *Francisella tularensis*).

Ramam and colleagues described a combination of 3 drugs, one of which was GM, that was effective in treating actinomycotic mycetomas in 7 patients [27]. Walker and Macaraeg reported a case of neonatal sepsis due to *C. perfringens* that was successfully treated with GM [28]. GM monotherapy was as effective as doxycycline (DOX) monotherapy for the treatment of plague, where GM 2.5 was used to treat plague caused by *Y. pestis* [29]. In an intentional (biological weapon) release setting, GM was recommended by the Working Group on Civilian Biodefense to treat tularemia and pneumonic plague (caused by *Y. pestis*) [30].

The disease treatment conditions include appendicitis, cat scratch disease, diarrhea, diverticulitis, female genital infection, uterine infection, peripartum and postnatal infection, malignant otitis externa, MD, NEC in fetus or newborn, osteomyelitis, PID, CF, and decubitus ulcer.

Intratympanic (IT) therapy with aminoglycosides (streptomycin) for MD was first described by Schuknecht in 1957 [31]. A meta-analysis published in 2004 by Cohen-Kerem et al. found that this treatment appeared to be effective in the relief of vertigo and that ototoxicity was unlikely to be a major side effect [32]. Intratympanically administered GM (ITG) has been used successfully [33-36]. Local ITG was effective in treating disabling MD in 15 of 16 patients [36]. Rauch and Oas reported an overall success rate of 65% (success minus relapse) following ITG in patients with intractable MD [33]. Other aminoglycoside antibiotics have been used in patients with severe disabling MD to ablate vestibular function and thus prevent recurrent episodes of vertigo [34, 35]. Chandler reported a high mortality rate in malignant external otitis secondary to *Pseudomonas* spp. and that it should be aggressively treated with parenteral aminoglycosides, such as GM, in combination with carbenicillin, ticarcillin, mezlocillin, or piperacillin [37].

Standard antibiotic therapy for appendicitis includes an aminoglycoside, commonly GM, in combination with clindamycin (CDM).

In recent years, several trials have compared this "gold standard" combination with other antibiotics, producing similar results. Treatment for appendicitis should encompass GN and anaerobic bacteria [15]. Hill et al. reported that metronidazole (MTD) in combination with GM and cholestyramine was effective in the treatment of persistent dehydrating diarrhea in infants [38]. In a double-blind randomized trial, 68 children with persistent diarrhea were randomized to placebo or GM for 6 days. No adverse effects were noted with GM therapy [39]. Similar results have been reported [40]. The use of GM for child and infantile diarrhea is controversial. The use of oral antibiotics (GM, kanamycin, and vancomycin) in the prevention of NEC reduces the incidence of NEC in low–birth weight infants, but concerns of adverse outcomes, including the development of resistant organisms, have not been adequately addressed. Rege reported that GM in combination with CDM or MTD was used successfully to treat complications from diverticulitis [41]. Hemsell et al. reported that meropenem monotherapy was as effective as the combination of CDM plus GM in the treatment of acute gynecologic and obstetric pelvic infection [42].

Harding et al. reported that a combination of GM and CDM, chloramphenicol, or ticarcillin were equally effective in the treatment of intra-abdominal and female genital tract sepsis [43]. One of the regimens recommended by the Centers for Disease Control and Prevention for the treatment of PID is CDM plus GM. In a randomized trial (n = 130) that compared the combination regimens of CDM plus GM and cefoxitin plus DOX for the treatment of PID, Walters and Gibbs found no significant differences in efficacy or adverse events [44].

Mitra et al. reported that combination therapy with once-daily GM was as safe and effective as combination therapy involving thrice-daily GM. Cure rates ranged from 88% to 94% in peripartum infection of the uterus and postnatal infection [45]. Studies from the 1990s reported that GM–collagen sponges were an effective means of achieving a rapid initial and high peak concentration of GM at the site of application. It was reported to be an efficacious adjuvant treatment in osteomyelitis [46, 47]. No large-scale studies compared the efficacy of GM–collagen sponges and GM-polymethyl-methacrylate during that decade.

GM in combination with ticarcillin-clavulanate was recommended as the regimen of choice in CF patients with pulmonary infections caused by *Haemophilus influenzae* and *Staph. aureus* [48].

Concerning decubitus ulcer, Anon reported that topical application of GM could be used to treat pressure sores [1]. The role of GM in relation to other standard therapies for this indication has not been determined.

The disease prophylaxis conditions include prophylaxis of postoperative infection of the nervous system, eye surgery, tympanostomy, postoperative infection in head and neck-related surgery, bacterial endocarditis, neutropenic status, burns, and cholestasis.

Limited data suggest that GM prophylaxis in combination with vancomycin reduces the incidence of postoperative neurosurgical wound infections [49]. Baker and Chole reported that topical GM ophthalmic solution applied as otic drops before and after tympanostomy with tube placement for otitis media was effective in preventing purulent otorrhea in the early postoperative period [50]. Topical GM is recommended for the prevention of wound infections and sepsis associated with ophthalmic surgery.

According to the guidelines of the American Heart Association, GM was recommended for prophylaxis of bacterial endocarditis, but that is currently not the case [41]. In head and neck surgical procedures that involve an incision through the oral or pharyngeal mucosa, the recommended antibiotic prophylaxis is cefazolin or the combination of CDM and GM [51]. GM plays a role in treating neutropenic fever. GM plus piperacillin was compared to imipenem in the treatment of febrile neutropenia in 252 cancer patients. At the end of treatment, the cure rate for imipenem was 55% and that for piperacillin plus GM was 53% [52]. GM has been recommended as an adjunct treatment option for empiric therapy of febrile neutropenia [53]. Combination therapy of GM and other antibiotics, including third-generation cephalosporins or antipseudomonal PENs, is effective for empiric treatment of febrile neutropenic patients [52, 54]. Once-daily GM was used effectively with additional antibiotics as empiric therapy for febrile neutropenia in children [55]. Both topical and parenteral GM were proven effective in increasing the rate of survival in burn patients with septicemia [56-58]. Adjusting GM dosages based on serum concentrations of GM was demonstrated to increase the rate of survival to burn patients[59, 60]. Anon reported that oral GM was used to prevent cholestasis in a small group of infants receiving hyperalimentation [1].

As the clinical data were limited, the use of GM for these non–FDA-approved labeling indications was controversial.

However, clinical studies in this field over the past decade have reported fair responses in the accumulated clinical experiences of GM; therefore, the use of GM in the above clinical conditions has been accepted.

Section 2. Medicinal Application of GM Today and in the Future

Over the last 50 years, GM was sometimes used for non–FDA-approved labeling indications because of bad clinical response to traditional treatment, the availability of preliminary results only (e.g., the results of clinical experience or from animal studies but not approved by the FDA), and low medical cost.

Due to limited evidence-based information, the use of GM for such indications was controversial. As clinical studies from the past 10 years have reported fair response to the accumulative clinical experiences of GM, it remains an important option for the above clinical conditions. We have reviewed the literature from the past 10 years, and have summarized the clinical conditions in Table 2. We have divided the indications for GM according to dosage form, and describe the indications and review articles in accordance to this division in the following sections.

Parenteral GM

GM had been widely used clinically since 1971. Parenteral GM may be used in 6 new conditions.

A. Bacteremia

1. Staphylococcus Saprophyticus Bacteremia

Staph. saprophyticus is generally susceptible to most antibiotics, including penicillin [61]. Forrest et al. demonstrated significantly high failure rates for single-dose penicillin therapy [61]. In our clinical experience, GM is one option that can be used to treat *Staph. saprophyticus* infection [62].

2. Bartonella Quintana Bacteremia

Bartonella quintana infection of humans was first described during World War I as being responsible for trench fever [63]. Recent reports have indicated a reemergence of *B. quintana* infections among the homeless population in cities in both Europe and the US [64, 65].

Recently, Foucault et al. retrospectively reviewed the data for bacteremic patients and found that only those who were treated with a combination of DOX and GM were cured, while those treated with beta-lactams or DOX alone were not [66].

Table 2. Medicinal application of GM today and in the future

Administration	Type	Indications
Parenteral	Bacteremia	*Staphylococcus saprophyticus* bacteremia *Bartonella quintana* bacteremia
	Neonatal sepsis	
	Gynecological infection	Intrapartum chorioamnionitis
	Eye surgery	Cataract surgery
	Coagulation	Effects of GM on platelet aggregation and blood coagulation
	Intratympanic therapy	Ménière's disease Preoperative vestibular ablation in
Lavage	Postoperative prophylaxis	Intra-abdominal infections
	Nasal infection	Pediatric chronic rhinosinusitis
GM–collagen sponge	Surgical site infection	Colorectal surgical site infection Anal fistula surgical site infection
		Pilonidal sinus wound infection
		Sternal wound infection
		Hidradenitis suppurativa
	Diabetic foot infections	
Topical	Cutaneous leishmaniasis	
	Prophylactic therapy	Peritoneal dialysis catheter exit site infections and peritonitis in uremia
GM-loaded cement spacers	Infected arthroplasty	
Nebulized	Decrease local infection	Decrease local infection in non-cystic fibrosis bronchiectasis
Oral GM	Decrease colonization rate	Carbapenem-resistant *Klebsiella pneumoniae* carriage
	Systemic diseases	Brucellosis
		Plague

To confirm those preliminary retrospective results, Foucault et al. conducted a randomized clinical trial from January 1, 2001 to April 1, 2002, and demonstrated the efficiency of the combination of DOX and GM in eradicating *B. quintana* bacteremia. The efficiency of this combination in eradicating *B. quintana* bacteremia may prevent the occurrence of *B. quintana* endocarditis efficiently [67].

B. Neonatal Sepsis

Neonatal sepsis is a life-threatening infection of the newborn that rarely occurs as late as 3 months of age. It is rarely viral or fungal and is often caused by organisms usually present in the maternal perineal flora. Signs of early-onset neonatal sepsis (EOS) are nonspecific, and prompt treatment with antibiotics has been shown to reduce mortality [68, 69]. Although not evaluated in appropriately powered clinical trials, the combination of a GM and ampicillin (AMP) or PEN has remained the treatment of choice for EOS in many nurseries worldwide [69, 70]. According Metsvaht et al., AMP and PEN combined with GM have similar effectiveness in the empiric treatment of suspected EOS [71]. Sepsis in the neonatal period is a major cause of child mortality in low-income countries. Appropriate community-based therapy in such situations is undefined. Zaidi et al. compared the failure rates of 3 clinic-based antibiotic regimens in 0–59-day-old infants with possible serious bacterial infection whose families refused hospitalization in Karachi communities and reported high neonatal mortality rates of >45/1000 live births [72]. The study found that treatment failure was significantly higher with trimethoprim-sulfamethoxazole (TMP-SMX)-GM as compared with PEN-GM. There were no significant differences when ceftriaxone was compared with PEN-GM. Outpatient therapy with injectable antibiotics is an effective option when hospitalization of sick infants is unfeasible. Procaine PEN-GM was superior to TMP-SMX-GM. Ceftriaxone is more expensive, and may be less effective [72]. The above studies suggest that PEN or AMP plus GM might be a preferred empirical regimen in neonatal sepsis as compared to other antibiotics. However, limited sample sizes and poor evidence suggest that further research is required to support this conclusion.

C. Gynecological Infection

Inflammation of the fetal membranes is termed chorioamnionitis. This can be associated with prolonged or premature rupture of the membranes or a primary cause of premature labor. The prevalence is about 50% of premature deliveries.

It is commonly associated with an ascending infection caused by organisms from the normal vaginal flora. Microorganisms are recognized by pattern recognition receptors (e.g., Toll-like receptors), which in turn elicit the release of inflammatory chemokines and cytokines. In a retrospective cohort study of preterm infants (<30-week gestation), Nasef and colleagues found that chorioamnionitis was associated with motor, cognitive, and language developmental delay [73].

Intrapartum treatment with AMP and GM reduces maternal febrile morbidity and length of stay and neonatal sepsis and length of stay when compared with postpartum treatment alone [74], although GM is classified as category D according to the pregnancy categories of both the US FDA and the Australian Drug Evaluation Committee. Extrapolated peak umbilical cord serum levels of GM were closer to ideal neonatal levels when treatment involved daily GM rather than 8-hour GM [45]. Treatment efficacy was equal when treatment involved daily GM and twice-daily CDM as compared with 8-hour GM and 8-hour CDM [75].

Lyell and colleagues conducted a randomized double-blind trial at the Labor and Delivery Unit at Lucile Packard Children's Hospital at the Stanford University Medical Center.

Treatment success was equal between groups (94% daily GM vs. 89% 8-hour GM, p = 0.53). They concluded that daily GM appeared to be as effective as 8-hour GM for the treatment of intrapartum chorioamnionitis without differences in maternal or neonatal morbidities [76]. Mitra et al. reported that combination therapy with once-daily GM was as safe and effective as combination therapy with thrice-daily GM. Cure rates ranged from 88% to 94% in peripartum infection of the uterus and postnatal infection [45]. However, a much larger study is needed to determine whether one regimen is superior to the other.

D. Ocular Infection

Phacoemulsification with intraocular lens implantation is currently the most common ophthalmic surgical procedure because of the high incidence of cataract; its combination with surgical advances makes modern cataract surgery highly successful and easy to perform as an outpatient procedure.

Despite advances in surgical techniques, endophthalmitis continues to be a sight-threatening complication of cataract surgery [77], and perioperative antibiotic prophylaxis may reduce the risk for endophthalmitis [78, 79].

Their prospective study enrolled 60 patients scheduled to undergo phacoemulsification surgery.

There was no significant difference between the anterior chamber cells of the treatment groups at 1 day and 1 week after surgery (p = 0.50 and 0.328, respectively). However, there were significantly fewer anterior chamber cells in the IC TA group than in the topical group 1 month post-operation (p = 0.006). No significant between-group difference in mean best-corrected visual acuity or intraocular pressure was noted at any time point (p > 0.05). No adverse effects or endophthalmitis were observed. Therefore, IC TA and GM appear to be a promising treatment option for the control of postoperative inflammation following cataract surgery.

Although IC TA and GM injections might be a useful strategy against endophthalmitis resulting from cataract surgery, subconjunctival injection resulted in more pain and was hence less acceptable to patients. Ahmed et al. used povidone iodine drops instead of subconjunctival injection of dexamethasone and GM combination at the end of phacoemulsification cataract surgery [80].

The anti-inflammatory and anti-infective effects and visual outcome were similar in both groups. IC TA and GM injections following cataract surgery resolved the issue of patient compliance, and 5% povidone iodine drop usage at the end of phacoemulsification surgery prevented pain and alleviated the patients' fears of subconjunctival injection. The preferred regimen should be determined according to a case-by-case basis. *Staphylococcus aureus* is an important and frequent cause of acute-onset endophthalmitis [81]. This bacterium is most commonly encountered after cataract surgery and often is associated with poor outcome [82, 83].

Therefore, in addition to IC TA and GM injections following cataract surgery to prevent postoperative endophthalmitis, some ophthalmic surgeons choose a vancomycin plus GM regimen instead [84]. Following a prospective randomized controlled trial (RCT), James et al. reported that there was increased central retinal thickness, which caused significantly reduced contrast sensitivity in those treated patients, but no statistically significant increase in macular thickness [85].

E. Effect on Coagulation

Aminoglycoside antibiotics, including GM, affect platelet aggregation and blood coagulation. Chen et al. reported that GM inhibited platelet aggregation, which contributed to whole blood clotting disorder.

GM might inhibit platelet aggregation by blocking the activation and release of some factor and likely by inhibiting endogenous clotting factor as well [86].

F. Intratympanic Therapy

The typical symptoms of MD can be managed using medical therapy that allows control of the disease in as many as two-thirds of patients [87]. An ablative approach is recommended when treatment cannot reduce the recurrent spells of vertigo. The advent of less invasive procedures, such as IT therapies, has greatly changed the treatment approach to refractory MD.

1. Ménière's Disease

For many years, GM was used for a predetermined duration until signs of ototoxicity developed [88-90]. The use of steroids for the treatment of MD was primarily based on the theory of an immune-mediated origin of the disease [91]. Several articles on IT steroids for MD have reported positive [92] and negative results [93]. Medical treatment cannot control the symptoms in about 5–10% of MD patients, and these patients suffer from frequent and serious vertigo spells with vomiting, which considerably limits their quality of life. The ideal endpoint of GM treatment is difficult to establish. Casani et al. designed an open prospective study and demonstrated that a combination of GM and fibrin glue permitted a reduction in the number of administrations in patients with intractable unilateral MD [94]. Subsequently, Casani et al. designed another open, prospective randomized controlled study to determine the efficacy and safety of low-dose ITG as compared with IT dexamethasone (ITD) in patients with intractable unilateral MD. Sixty patients affected by definite unilateral MD were enrolled between January 1, 2007 and June 30, 2008. The study produced evidence that supported the hypothesis that IT delivery of low-dose GM was a relatively safe and effective therapy for the treatment of intractable MD, providing superior vertigo control as compared with ITD (ITG vs. ITD, 93.5% vs. 61%, respectively) and was associated with a very low incidence of hearing impairment (12.5%) [95]. Moreover, high-dose ITG was successful in achieving long-term control of vertigo for patients (n = 14) with intractable MD [96] (Hsieh, Lin et al. 2009).

Delgado and Peña designed a longitudinal prospective descriptive study of response to GM treatment in 71 patients who had been diagnosed with MD and treated medically for more than a year. The ITG injection protocol enabled effective vertigo control in most patients and represented a good alternative to more aggressive techniques for the treatment of MD that does not respond to medical treatment [97]. Postema et al. carried out a prospective randomized, placebo-controlled trial to investigate the efficacy of GM application in the treatment of unilateral MD. GM treatment resulted in a significant reduction in the scores for vertigo complaints and perceived aural fullness.

A small increase in hearing loss was recorded in the GM group. The treatment also reduced the severity of the perceived aural fullness. ITG is a relatively safe and efficient treatment for the reduction of complaints of vertigo attacks associated with MD. Conservative medical treatment is quite effective in eliminating symptoms in many patients with MD. ITG therapy is a treatment option for patients with intractable MD attempting to eliminate vertigo complaints while preserving their hearing. The study by Postema et al. supports the apparent effectiveness of ITG therapy in the relief of vertigo and the notion that ototoxicity is unlikely to be a major side effect [98]. Perez and Rama-Lopez analyzed the effects of ITG injections on vestibular function in 33 patients with unilateral MD that had been unresponsive to medical therapy for at least 1 year.

After treatment, both the time constant of the vestibulo-ocular reflex (VOR) after rotation towards the treated side and the gain in the sinusoidal harmonic acceleration test were significantly reduced. These reductions were in accordance with the number of additional signs observed upon bedside examination at the end of the treatment. The changes observed in the VOR correlated well with the results of the bedside examination of vestibular function, which in turn reflected the damage induced by ITG injection [99]. Stokroos and Kingma designed a prospective double-blind randomized clinical trial of ITG vs. IT buffer solution (placebo) in patients with established active MD in the affected ear. ITG is a safe and efficient treatment for the vertiginous spells associated with MD. When applied early in the course of the disease, it may prevent some of the sensorineural hearing deterioration associated with it [100].

2. Preoperative Vestibular Ablation with GM

An acute vestibular lesion causes the well-known symptoms of vestibular loss, featuring vertigo, nausea, and ataxia. By way of central nervous compensation and recalibration, most symptoms subside over weeks to months. This process has been demonstrated as being dependent on cerebellar function [101].

Magnusson et al. reported the experience of ablating vestibular function accompanied by a vestibular prehabilitation program (PREHAB) in advance of surgery to prevent postoperative vertigo and vestibular loss symptoms when recovering from the intracranial surgery.

Twelve patients with pontine angle tumors but with near normal vestibular function were treated with ITG in combination with vestibular PREHAB to achieve preoperative vestibular ablation and compensation.

Preoperative GM in combination with vestibular PREHAB presents the possibility of reducing postoperative malaise and speeded up recovery, and may be used for patients undergoing such surgery when there is remaining vestibular function. The approach of Magnusson and colleagues, which combined vestibular PREHAB with pre-surgery GM ablation of vestibular function, suggests the possibility of reducing morbidity in patients in whom intracranial surgery will induce acute vestibular loss [102].

The literature reveals that vestibular PREHAB and GM before schwannoma surgery may improve long-term postural function. Patients scheduled for vestibular schwannoma surgery are subject to challenging rehabilitation processes partly due to the intracranial surgery, but also because of the effects of acute unilateral vestibular deafferentation (uVD).

Recently, a treatment procedure was reported in which patients with remnant vestibular function before surgery were ablated by the administration of GM in the middle ear [103]. As performed in vestibular schwannoma surgery, uVD results in chronic vestibular deficit, though most of the insufficiency can be compensated by other sensory input. By carrying out vestibular PREHAB before surgery, motor adaptation processes can be instigated before the actual lesion is produced.

The adaptation processes of the altered sensory input could be affected if the vestibular ablation and surgery were separated early by pretreating patients with remaining vestibular function with GM. Tjernström et al. assessed recordings made with vibratory proprioceptive stimulation before and after surgery in patients with varying vestibular function with the specific aim of investigating whether presurgical deafferentation and sensory training would also affect post-surgery postural control in the longer term, which was up to 6 months after surgery in their report.

The results indicated that pretreating patients who have remaining vestibular function with GM before ablative surgery benefits not only postoperative wellbeing as previously described, but also the long-term learning of how to withstand perturbed postural control, i.e., the ability to cope with sensory conflicts.

The findings indicate a rationale for treating even more patients scheduled for vestibular schwannoma surgery with vestibular PREHAB and GM, at least when no hearing conservation is required [104].

Excluding its empirical use for treatment of the febrile neutropenic patient or patients with serious nosocomial infection due to its broad spectrum of bactericidal activity against common and unusual *Enterobacteriaceae, P. aeruginosa*, and staphylococci, parenteral GM can be used in many situations.

In addition, because of the widespread use of broad-spectrum beta-lactam antibiotics and fluoroquinolones, there has been a significant increase in the emergence of multidrug-resistant bacteria, such as *B. quintana*, which often require treatment with a synergistic combination of GM with another antibiotic. GM might also inhibit platelet aggregation by blocking the activation and release of some factor, and likely by inhibiting endogenous clotting factor as well [86]. GM is available in ophthalmic ointment and solution form to treat a variety of ophthalmic infections, including blepharitis, conjunctivitis, keratitis, and corneal ulcers, and is available as topical ointment or cream preparations to treat dermatologic infections such as impetigo contagiosa, acne, and seborrheic dermatitis. The use of IC TA and GM injections following cataract surgery can resolve the issue of patient compliance.

The dosage and dosage interval of GM is currently being studied. GM can be used more widely in the pediatric and gynecological fields. Daily GM appears to be as effective as 8-hour GM for the treatment of intrapartum chorioamnionitis without differences in maternal or neonatal morbidities.

ITG presents the possibility of reducing the severity of MD, and GM ablation of vestibular function might reduce morbidity in patients in whom intracranial surgery will induce acute vestibular loss.

Lavage with GM Solution

Typically, an antibiotic lavage consists of perioperative or peritoneal irrigation to prevent infectious diseases. According to the literature, there are 2 conditions in which GM solution would be effective.

A. Postoperative Prophylaxis

Many surgeons have adopted the use of peritoneal lavage in abdominal surgeries. Generally, this consists of peritoneal irrigation with a varied volume of 0.9% sodium chloride (normal saline). The effects of lavage have been widely studied for the management of patients with bacterial peritonitis, although the appropriate volume and carrier remain unclear, as does the benefit of including antibiotics or antiseptics.

1. Intra-Abdominal Infections

To reduce the morbidity and mortality of intra-abdominal infections, surgeons aim to isolate and control the source of contamination.

It has been proposed that lavage removes bacterial contamination and other materials that may promote bacterial proliferation and proinflammatory cytokines that may enhance local inflammation. The lavage may be combined with antibiotics to reduce bacterial survival further. In a prospective randomized study, Ruiz-Tovar et al. enrolled patients who had been diagnosed with colorectal neoplasm and who had planned to undergo elective curative surgery. The use of CDM-GM solution in peritoneal lavage was associated with a lower incidence of intra-abdominal abscesses and wound infections [105].

B. Nasal Infection

1. Pediatric Chronic Rhinosinusitis

The prospective, randomized, double-blind study of Wei et al. was designed to compare the efficacy and outcome of daily saline irrigation vs. saline/GM for treating chronic rhinosinusitis (CRS). The high tolerance, compliance, and effectiveness of once-daily intranasal GM irrigation supported its use as a first-line treatment for pediatric CRS before surgical intervention was considered [106].

Using GM solution in peritoneal lavage was associated with a lower incidence of intra-abdominal abscesses and wound infections. The use of GM solution in treating CRS was associated with higher quality of life.

GM–Collagen Sponge

GM–collagen sponges have been used since the 1990s; recent publications have reported their application in most surgical site and diabetic wound infections.

A. Surgical Site Infection

Surgical wound infections are the second most common healthcare-associated infection. Although usually localized to the incision site, surgical wound infections can also extend into adjacent deeper structures; thus, the term "surgical wound infection" has been replaced with the more accurate "surgical site infection" (SSI). SSIs may lead to prolonged hospital stay and increased morbidity, mortality, and hospital costs.

SSIs are the most common nosocomial infection among surgical patients, accounting for 38% of nosocomial infections.

It is estimated that SSIs develop in 2–5% of the more than 30 million patients who undergo surgical procedures each year (i.e., 1 out of every 24 patients who undergo inpatient surgery in the US has a postoperative SSI) [107, 108].

There are many general control measures to reduce SSI rates, including antimicrobial prophylaxis. Many surgeons believe that local use of antibiotics is a new essential method for postoperative reduction of wound complications.

The GM–collagen sponge, an implantable topical antibiotic agent, is a new technique for antibiotic prophylaxis in surgical wounds in addition to conventional intravenous (IV) antibiotics. It is approved for surgical implantation in 54 countries [109]. Since 1985, more than 1 million patients have been treated with the sponges. It was developed to prevent and treat wound infections by providing high GM concentrations locally, avoiding the high systemic concentrations associated with the risk of toxic adverse reactions, such as nephrotoxicity [110]. The collagen matrix of the sponge biodegrades and disappears within days to weeks. Pharmacokinetic data show that implantation of 1–5 sponges (corresponding to 130–650 mg GM) resulted in very high local tissue GM concentrations of 170–9000 µg/mm. These concentrations exceeded the minimum inhibitory concentrations (MIC) for many microorganisms. Systemic concentrations of GM, however, remained below 2 µg/mm 24 hours after implantation [111].

The high GM concentration in the wound achieved by local application of GM may be effective against bacteria that, based on their MIC, are normally considered resistant [110]. Several studies suggest that the sponge may be effective in the prevention and treatment of infections after general surgery [112-114]. In this literature review, we found that the GM–collagen sponge was used in at least 5 different SSIs, and the SSIs were caused by reduction of wound complications post-surgery

1. Colorectal SSI

In a single-center, nonblinded randomized trial, 221 patients who underwent colorectal surgery and received a sponge had 70% less SSI as compared with those who did not receive a sponge (18.4% vs. 5.6%, respectively; p < 0.01) [112]. Bennett-Guerrero et al. carried out a larger, multi-center randomized clinical trial in which 602 patients undergoing open or laparoscopically assisted colorectal surgery at 39 "US" sites received either 2 GM–collagen sponges above the fascia at the time of surgical closure (sponge group) or no intervention (control group).

Each sponge (10 cm × 10 cm) contained 280 mg collagen and 130 mg GM. The incidence of SSI was higher in the sponge group than in the control group (30% vs. 20.9%, p = 0.01). There was superficial SSI in 20.3% of patients in the sponge group and in 13.6% of patients in the control group (p = 0.03), and deep SSI in 8.3% and 6.0% of sponge and control group patients (p = 0.26), respectively. The authors concluded that the GM–collagen sponge was not effective for preventing SSI in patients who had undergone colorectal surgery; paradoxically, it appeared to result in significantly more SSIs [109].

2. Anal Fistula SSI

Endoanal advancement flap repair is widely used in sphincter-preserving surgery for anal fistula, but the high recurrence rate is a major problem. A possible cause of non-healing is local infection of the flap. Local application of the GM–collagen sponge has been used both to prevent and to treat surgical wound infection.

The study of Gustafsson and Graf was designed to evaluate whether local antibiotic treatment with the GM–collagen sponge improved healing after endoanal advancement flap repair for anal fistula. Eighty-three patients who underwent the procedure were randomized to surgery with (42 patients) or without (41 patients) application of the GM–collagen sponge beneath the flap. Patients were evaluated at 1–3 and 12 months after surgery for healing and/or recurrence. The overall healing rate with no recurrence at 1 year after surgery was 57%. Twenty-six of 42 patients randomized to the GM–collagen sponge healed primarily as compared with 21 of the 41 patients randomized to surgery only. The primary recurrence rate of endoanal advancement flap repair for anal fistula was 61 percent. Healing was not significantly improved by local application of the GM–collagen sponge [17].

3. Pilonidal Sinus Wound Infection

Pilonidal sinus is a common disease that leads to the substantial loss of many work hours, but treatment is variable and problematic. Excision and primary suture for pilonidal disease is associated with a high rate of wound infection and recurrences.

In the controlled, prospective, randomized double-blind single-center study of Yetim et al., 80 patients undergoing surgical treatment for pilonidal sinus were randomly assigned to 2 groups. Group 1 (control) received oral antibiotics for 7 days postoperation. In group 2, GM–collagen sponges were placed on the sacral fascia prior to wound closure, and these patients did not receive oral postoperative antibiotic therapy.

The patients in group 2 had significantly shorter mean wound healing time and hospital stay and significantly lower infection and recurrence rates than those in group 1. The authors concluded that the implantation of a GM–collagen sponge in the wound area in pilonidal sinus decreased the rate of infection and recurrence and shortened hospital stay [115].

Andersson et al. designed a randomized controlled study to analyze the effect of local application of a GM–collagen sponge in reducing the wound infection rate and recurrence after excision of pilonidal sinus and wound closure with primary midline suture. One hundred and sixty-one patients with symptomatic pilonidal disease underwent surgery at 11 hospitals, undergoing traditional wide excision of the sinus and all of its tracts.

All patients were randomized to filling of the cavity with a GM–collagen sponge before wound closure or to closure with no additional treatment. Patients who received prophylaxis in the form of the GM–collagen sponge had slightly fewer wounds with exudate at 2–4 days and 2 weeks of follow-up (2% vs. 10%, p = 0.051 and 57% vs. 65%, p = 0.325, respectively) and a slightly larger proportion of healed wounds at 3 months' follow-up (77% vs. 66%, p = 0.138).

There were no significant differences in the rates of wound infection, wound healing, or recurrences when a GM–collagen sponge was added to the surgical treatment of pilonidal disease with excision and primary midline suture. The study did not support the use of the GM–collagen sponge for the surgical treatment of pilonidal disease [116].

The controlled, multi-centre trial of Holzer et al. was designed to evaluate the efficacy of a new GM collagen fleece combined with primary closure (PC). The trial enrolled 103 patients. Fifty-one patients were randomized to GM fleece plus PC (genta group), and 52 patients to open treatment alone (open group). Two patients in genta group developed infection within the first 2 weeks, requiring reopening of the wound, with primary wound healing occurring in 73%. Failure of primary healing (27%) was usually due to seroma or spontaneous dehiscence, which subsequently healed. The combination of GM collagen fleece with PC resulted in a shorter healing period than the open technique, and without unwanted effects [117].

Excision and PC over GM-impregnated collagen is a cost-effective method of treating pilonidal sinuses, as it ensures faster healing, causes less pain, and its long-term recurrence rates are similar to other techniques. However, this approach is controversial.

Further larger quality-controlled studies are needed to prove the effectiveness of GM-impregnated collagen.

4. Sternal Wound Infection

In open cardiac surgery, sternal wound infection (SWI) continues to be one of the most serious postoperative complications, with significant associated costs, lengthened hospital stay, and increased mortality [118-120].

Although systemic antimicrobial prophylaxis is routinely administered, SWIs remain a major threat, leading surgeons to seek additional preventive measures. Prophylactic retrosternal placement of a GM–collagen sponge has been the subject of several recent clinical studies and is a matter of controversy.

The controlled, prospective, randomized, double-blind single-center study of Schimmer et al. was designed to investigate the efficacy of a retrosternal GM–collagen sponge in reducing sternal wound complications after cardiac surgery. The study enrolled 720 consecutive patients who underwent median sternotomy, assigning them to a control placebo group (collagen sponge) or an intervention group (GM–collagen sponge). The incidence of deep SWIs was 3.52% (control placebo group) vs. 0.56% (intervention group); p = 0.014. Treatment for all SWIs and deep SWIs was required for 26(control placebo group) and 33 patients(intervention group), respectively. Routine prophylactic retrosternal use of a GM–collagen sponge in patients undergoing cardiac surgery significantly reduced deep SWIs [121].

The single-blind, prospective RCT of Bennett-Guerrero et al. enrolled 1502 cardiac surgical patients at high risk for SWI. All patients were randomized to insertion of 2 GM–collagen sponges between the sternal halves at surgical closure (n = 753) vs. no intervention (control group: n = 749). The primary analysis found no significant difference in SWIs (superficial and deep). Among US cardiac surgery patients with diabetes, high body mass index, or both, the use of 2 GM–collagen sponges as compared with no intervention did not reduce the 90-day SWI rate [122].

Friberg's randomized, prospective double-blind trial was designed to evaluate the efficacy of GM–collagen sponges in SWI after cardiac surgery (sternotomy). At the end of the operation, immediately before sternal closure, 1950 patients were assigned to the treatment group (routine IV prophylaxis combined with sternal application of GM–collagen sponge) or the control group (IV isoxazolyl PEN alone). The incidence of any SWI was 4.3% in the treatment group and 9.0% in the control group (p < 0.001). Local GM reduced the incidence of SWI caused by all major clinically important microbiological agents, including coagulase-negative staphylococci (CoNS). Routine use of the described prophylaxis in all adult cardiac surgery patients was recommended [123].

The cost-effectiveness study of Friberg et al. aimed to evaluate the economic rationale for the use of GM collagen in everyday clinical practice. The study identified the high-risk groups that may have derived particular benefit. The study calculated the costs attributable to the SWI for each patient with SWI. Risk factors for SWI were identified and any heterogeneity of the effect of the prophylaxis was examined. The mean cost of a SWI was about 14500 Euros.

The positive net balance was even higher in high- risk groups. Assignment to the control group, overweight, diabetes, younger age, mammarian artery use, left ventricular ejection fraction < 35%, and longer operation time were independent risk factors for infection. The addition of local GM collagen to IV antibiotic prophylaxis was beneficial, i.e., it resulted in both lower costs and fewer wound infections [118].

Eklund et al. investigated whether locally administered GM would prevent SWIs in coronary artery bypass graft (CABG) surgery. They randomized 542 consecutive CABG patients to 2 groups: those who received a GM–collagen sponge under the sternum before closure (n = 272), and controls (n = 270). The subjects received routine IV antimicrobial prophylaxis and were followed-up for 3 months. The SWI rate was 4.0% (11/272) in the genta group and 5.9% (16/270) in the control group. The rates of mediastinitis were 1.1% (genta group) and 1.9% (control group).

No statistically significant difference was demonstrated between infection rates in the 2 groups. The data show that infection was reduced slightly in the genta group as compared with the control group, but the study population was too small to draw conclusions [124].

These studies provide evidence that supports the use of the GM–collagen sponge for the prevention of postoperative SWIs in patients undergoing cardiac surgery. However, additional large, high-quality RCTs are warranted to further elucidate this field.

5. Hidradenitis Suppurativa

Hidradenitis suppurativa (HS) is a chronic recurrent inflammatory disease of the apocrine sweat glands. The disease mainly affects the axillary and anogenital regions; it occurs in both sexes, with women being affected 3 times more frequently than men [125, 126].

Controversy remains regarding the appropriate treatment for HS. In the early stages, the disease is often treated with antibiotics and simple measures, such as usage of antiseptic substances, systemic antibiotics, absolute cessation of smoking, and limited incision and drainage [127].

Buimer and colleagues described a prospective randomized study on the use of GM–collagen sponge in the surgical treatment of HS and reported that enclosing a GM–collagen sponge after primary excision of HS reduced the number of complications 1 week post-operation.

Furthermore, the wound was completely healed within 2 months in 65% of the patients treated with GM–collagen sponge.

There was no effect on the long-term recurrence rate. Their results demonstrate that excision of hidradenitis lesions with PC over a GM–collagen sponge reduces the number of postoperative complications and results in a clean, fast-healing wound. The use of a GM–collagen sponge with excision and PC was recommended. [128].

B. Diabetic Foot Infections

The pilot study of Lipsky and associates aimed to determine the safety and potential benefit of the addition of a topical GM–collagen sponge to the standard of care (systemic antibiotic therapy plus standard diabetic wound management) for treating diabetic foot infections of moderate severity. Fifty-six patients with moderately infected diabetic foot ulcers were randomized in a 2:1 ratio to receive standard of care plus a GM–collagen sponge or standard of care only for up to 28 days. On treatment day 7, they noted clinical cure in the treatment patients and 3 control patients ($p = 0.017$).

However, for evaluable patients at the test-of-cure visit, there was a significantly higher proportion of patients in the treatment group with clinical cure than the control group (100.0% vs. 70.0%, respectively; $p = 0.024$). Patients in the treatment group also had a higher rate of eradication of baseline pathogens at all visits ($p \leq 0.038$) and a reduced time to pathogen eradication ($p < 0.001$). They reported that topical application of the GM–collagen sponge appeared safe and might improve clinical and microbiological outcomes of diabetic foot infections of moderate severity when combined with standard of care. The pilot data suggested that a larger trial of this treatment was warranted [129].

Topical GM

This dosage form is the earliest form in which GM was applied; most of the conditions were related to wound care. The literature contains 2 clinical situations that provided good clinical evidence for this use of GM.

A. Cutaneous Leishmaniasis

Leishmania, a genus of trypanosomatid protozoa, is endemic in 98 countries or territories worldwide, and infection is transmitted by the bite of a female sandfly. The annual incidence of cutaneous leishmaniasis (CL) globally is 1.0–1.5 million cases [130]. There are several therapeutic options, but none is optimal [131]. CL is a disfiguring disease that leaves clinicians in a quandary: leave patients untreated or engage in a complex or toxic treatment. Topical treatment of CL is a practical and safe option. CL results from the parasitization of skin macrophages and generally manifests as a papule that enlarges to a nodule that often ulcerates over a period of 1–3 months. A variety of therapies for CL has been reviewed. Clearly, there remains a need for a treatment that is simple, efficacious, and with an acceptable side effect profile. One non-systemic treatment is the topical application of paromomycin-containing creams.

Ben Salah et al. developed a cream called WR279,396 that contained 15% paromomycin sulfate plus 0.5% GM sulfate in a complex base to aid drug penetration, and conducted a randomized, vehicle-controlled phase 3 trial of topical treatments containing 15% paromomycin with and without 0.5% GM for CL. The rate of cure of the index lesion was 81% for paromomycin alone and 58% for the vehicle control (p < 0.001). Mild to moderate application site reactions were more frequent in the paromomycin groups than in the vehicle-control group. The trial provided evidence of the efficacy of paromomycin-GM and paromomycin alone for ulcerative *L. major* disease. It also demonstrated that the efficacy of either of 2 creams containing 15% paromomycin with and without 0.5% GM was superior to that of a vehicle-control cream for treating ulcerative CL caused by *L. major* in Tunisia. The study observed no advantage following the addition of GM [132].

B. Prophylactic Therapy

1. PD Catheter Exit Site Infections and Peritonitis in Uremia

Peritonitis is the major cause of PD technique failure. Prophylactic topical antibiotics have been reported to reduce PD catheter exit site infections (ESIs) and peritonitis rates. Davenport et al. reviewed the effect of ESIs and peritonitis between 2005 and 2008. Topical antibiotics were reported to reduce both ESI and peritonitis rates in controlled trials, and although this review of routine clinical practice determined that topical mupirocin reduced overall ESI rates and that both mupirocin and GM reduced *Staph. aureus* ESIs, neither reduced overall peritonitis rates [133].

Ointment containing GM was found to be safe and effective for treating *L. major* CL, and has great potential as inexpensive topical therapy for CL and as prophylactic therapy for PD ESIs and peritonitis.

GM-Loaded Cement Spacers

Surgeons have used GM-containing materials, such as GM sponges, in surgical sites for many years, and we reviewed the literature to summarize these clinical applications.

PJI is one of the most frequent complications in total hip arthroplasty and total knee arthroplasty, and is often associated with significant morbidity and increased medical costs [134]. Most PJIs are caused by gram-positive pathogens. Staphylococci (including *Staph. aureus* and CoNS) and streptococci are among the most common organisms, which constitute 65–85% of all isolates. GN bacteria, which are less commonly involved in PJI, constitute 6–23% of all isolates [135-138]. Although there have been numerous reports regarding the treatment of PJI, specific descriptions of GN PJIs are limited. While comprising a relatively minor proportion of all PJIs, GN infections are of significant clinical importance because treatment of such infections is considered more complicated due to the virulence of the organisms, their growing resistance to antimicrobial agents, and the comorbid conditions of patients [139-141].

A. Infected Arthroplasty

The current standard surgical procedure in managing prosthetic hip infections is staged exchange arthroplasty, which involves the removal of all components by thorough debridement of the infected tissues, followed by a period of antibiotic treatment and reimplantation of a new prosthesis at a later stage [142].

The use of antibiotic-loaded cement spacers (ALCS) to treat PJIs has gained popularity over the recent decades, with reported infection eradication rates ranging from 90% to 100% [143-146]. ALCS not only function as a temporary hip joint implant, but can also be utilized for direct local antibiotic delivery [137]. Vancomycin plus GM is the preferred regimen in the composition of ALCS. Both drugs possess a narrow therapeutic index and require therapeutic drug monitoring in generic IV administration. Therefore, the utilization of this regimen raises the concern of systemic safety.

Another study by Springer and colleagues reported that no patient exhibited any clinical evidence of acute renal insufficiency, failure, or other systemic side effects of GM. Using high-dose vancomycin and GM antibiotic spacers to treat patients with infected total knee arthroplasty appeared clinically safe [147].

Nebulized GM

Nebulized antibiotics were used throughout the 1980s, but the clinical response at the time was inadequate.

Throughout the past decade, GM was nebulized to decrease bacterial load and local infection in non-CF bronchiectasis.

A. Decreased Bacterial Load and Local Infection in Non-CF Bronchiectasis

Bronchiectasis is a chronic debilitating disease with few evidence-based long-term treatments. Murray and colleagues conducted an RCT to assess the efficacy of nebulized GM therapy in patients with non-CF bronchiectasis and reported that regular long-term nebulized GM was of significant benefit in non-CF bronchiectasis, but that continuous treatment was required to ensure ongoing efficacy. Such infections are difficult to eradicate with systemic antibiotics because the structural abnormalities in the bronchial wall reduce their bactericidal effect at this level [148]. Inhaled GM can reduce bacterial load and local infection in both CF and non-CF bronchiectasis.

Oral GM

The oral form of GM is used for clinical conditions. We have summarized the following:

A. Decreased Colonization Rate

1. Eradication of Carbapenem-Resistant *K. Pneumoniae* Carriage by Selective Digestive Decontamination

The emergence of *K. pneumoniae* carbapenemase has been of particular concern because it resides on transmissible plasmids, and the carbapenem-resistant *K. pneumoniae* (CRKP) harboring these enzymes are resistant to almost all available antimicrobial agents [148, 149]. Selective digestive decontamination (SDD) aims to eradicate abnormal aerobic GN bacteria while preserving anaerobic bacteria in the gastrointestinal tract through the use of nonabsorbable, enterally administered antibiotics (e.g., polymyxin E and tobramycin). Saidel-Odes and associates designed a randomized, double-blind, placebo-controlled study to assess the effectiveness of SDD for eradicating CRKP oropharyngeal and gastrointestinal carriage [150]. They reported that 3 days after receiving oral GM and polymyxin E gel and oral solutions of GM and polymyxin E, the throat cultures for CRKP in the SDD arm became negative (p < 0.0001). SDD of the digestive tract is the only evidence-based approach that prevents infection and mortality in critically ill patients hospitalized in the intensive care unit.

As an enteral antimicrobial approach, an SDD regimen containing GM could be a suitable decolonization therapy for selected patients colonized with CRKP, such as transplant recipients or immunocompromised patients pending chemotherapy, and patients who require major intestinal or oropharyngeal surgery [150].

B. Systemic Diseases

Brucellosis is an important public health problem worldwide [151, 152]. When GM and DOX were used for 7 and 45 days, respectively, the rates of success in 3 studies were between 86% and 94.8% [153-155]. Plague is a natural infection of rodents caused by the bacterium *Y. pestis*, and is transmitted to humans by rodent flea bites, and less commonly, from person to person by respiratory droplets from coughing patients [156, 157]. Over the past 50 years, the antibiotics of choice for the treatment of plague, including streptomycin, chloramphenicol, and tetracycline, have mostly become outdated. GM was effective against *Y. pestis* in vitro [158] and in experimental animal infections [159]. We have reviewed new studies on the clinical applications of GM for these 2 systemic diseases.

1. Human Brucellosis

The efficacy of 5-day GM plus 8-week DOX administration was 100% in children with brucellosis [160]. As the efficacy of this regimen in adult brucellosis had not been determined, Roushan and associates aimed to compare the efficacy of 5-day GM plus 8-week DOX vs. 2-week streptomycin plus 45-day DOX in the treatment of human brucellosis. They found that the rate of success of the 5-day GM plus 8-week DOX treatment (95.12%) was not significantly superior to that of 2-week streptomycin plus 45-day DOX (89%).

The results also showed that the efficacy of the 5-day GM plus 8-week DOX treatment was not superior to that of 2-week streptomycin plus 45-day DOX [161].

2. Plague

A recent retrospective analysis of human cases of plague was recently reported [162], but there has not been a controlled prospective assessment of human infection.

Mwengee et al. conducted their trial to test the efficacy and safety of GM for the plague. GM and DOX were effective therapies for adult and pediatric plague, with high rates of favorable responses and low rates of adverse events [29].

Despite the glut of newly developed antibiotics in the current century, GM still plays a role in medicinal applications.

As the availability of less toxic agents means that it is usually not used alone to treat staphylococcal infections, GM possesses appreciable activity against staphylococci.

By contrast, a beta-lactam antibiotic or vancomycin is often combined with GM to treat serious staphylococcal infections to take advantage of their synergistic actions and the increased rate of bactericidal action. GM is commonly used in combination with cell wall–active agents such as beta-lactams and vancomycin in the therapy of enterococcal endocarditis.

As mentioned previously, GM may be used for inhalational therapy, primarily in the management of *P. aeruginosa* in CF patients. GM is available in ophthalmic ointment and solution form to treat a variety of ophthalmic infections, including blepharitis, conjunctivitis, keratitis, and corneal ulcers, and is available as topical ointment or cream preparations to treat dermatologic infections such as impetigo contagiosa, acne, and seborrheic dermatitis.

GM has been used in combination with paromomycin to treat exotic infections caused by *F. tularensis* (tularemia), *Y. pestis* (plague), and *Brucella* spp. (brucellosis). This antibiotic produces good effects in different dosage forms, including in sponge, cement, and solution form.

CONCLUSION

From this literature review, it is clear that there are many medicinal applications for GM, and the antibiotic remains a crucial element in the treatment of infectious diseases.

To reduce the development of GM-resistant bacteria and to maintain its effectiveness, GM should be used only to treat or prevent infections proven or strongly suspected as being caused by susceptible bacteria. New strategies such as single daily dosing and applications to non–FDA-approved labeling indications have the potential to decrease cost and toxicity while improving efficiency. In the future, GM will be more widely used in combination therapy and applied to medical materials for clinical application, and most of those indications have yet to be approved by the FDA. It would now be appropriate to carry out a definitive, suitably powered study of the clinical applications of GM, especially in terms of its effectiveness, safety, and cost.

REFERENCES

[1]   A. (1996). The choice of antibacterial drugs. *The Medical Letter*, 38, 25-34.

[2]   L, R. J. (1975). Two Children with Pseudomonas Osteomyelitis: The Paucity of Systemic Symptoms May Lead to Delay in Diagnosis. *Clinical Pediatrics*, 14, 288-291.

[3]   M, P. O. and K, T. B. and M, A. (1976). Comparison of tobramycin and gentamicin in the treatment of complicated urinary tract infections. *Journal of Infectious Diseases*, 134, S150-S152.

[4]   W, B. D. and G, L. O. (1976). A randomized, comparative study of tobramycin and gentamicin in treatment of acute urinary tract infections. *Journal of Infectious Diseases*, 134, S146-S149.

[5]   Information, P., *Gentamicin sulfate topical cream, ointment.* Taro Pharmaceuticals Inc, Hawthorne, NY. 2004.

[6]   S, G. (1974). Proteus endophthalmitis. *Archives of ophthalmology*, 91, 419.

[7]   H, K. and H, S. E. (1976). Intraventricular treatment of Serratia marcescens meningitis with gentamicin: pharmacokinetic studies of GM concentration in one case. *Scandinavian Journal of Infectious Diseases*, 8, 57-60.

[8]   K, F. A. and K, A. R. (1973). Serratia marcescens endocarditis. *Annals of Internal Medicine,* 79, 454-454.

[9]   T, A. R., et al. (2004). Practice guidelines for the management of bacterial meningitis. *Clinical infectious diseases,* 39, 1267-1284.

[10] S, A. F. and F, W. E. (1974). Intracisternal and intrathecal injections of gentamicin in Enterobacter meningitis. *Archives of Internal Medicine*, 134, 738.

[11] U, N., et al. (1980). Meningitis due to Haemophilus influenzae type b resistant to ampicillin and chloramphenicol. *The Journal of pediatrics*, 97, 421.

[12] T, P. and L, M. and P, L. (1975). Successful treatment of Pseudomonas meningitis and septicemia in a leukemic neutropenic adult. *American journal of clinical pathology*, 63, 135-141.

[13] P, G. A. and R, H. (1974). Bacterial endophthalmitis: treatment with intraocular injection of GM and dexamethasone. *Archives of Ophthalmology*, 91, 416-418.

[14] G, S. (1974). Proteus endophthalmitis. *Archives of Ophthalmology*, 91, 419.

[15] M, G. L. and D, R. G. and B, J. E., *Principles and Practice of Infectious Diseases*. 3rd ed. 1990, New York: Churchill Livingstone.

[16] B, L. M., et al. (2005). Infective Endocarditis Diagnosis, Antimicrobial Therapy, and Management of Complications: A Statement for Healthcare Professionals From the Committee on Rheumatic Fever, Endocarditis, and Kawasaki Disease, Council on Cardiovascular Disease in the Young, and the Councils on Clinical Cardiology, Stroke, and Cardiovascular Surgery and Anesthesia, American Heart Association: Endorsed by the Infectious Diseases Society of America. *Circulation*, 111, e394-e434.

[17] G, U. M. and G, W. (2006). Randomized clinical trial of local gentamicin–collagen treatment in advancement flap repair for anal fistula. *British journal of surgery*, 93, 1202-1207.

[18] S, S. (1984). Gentamicin injection: Single daily dose in urinary tract infections. *Current Therapeutic Research, Clinical and Experimental*, 35, 937-943.

[19] Z, B. J. and S, D. S. (1982). Hot tub folliculitis: a clinical syndrome. *Western Journal of Medicine*, 137, 191-194.

[20] C, C. F. D. (1983). An outbreak of Pseudomonas folliculitis associated with a waterslide--Utah. *Morbidity and Mortality Weekly Report*, 32, 425-427.

[21] C, C. F. D. (1982). Otitis due to Pseudomonas aeruginosa serotype 0:10 associated with a mobile redwood hot tub system--North Carolina. *Morbidity and Mortality Weekly Report.*, 31, 541-542.

[22] S, C. and S, A. (1973). Gentamicin therapy of severe infections. *Acta Pathologica Microbiologica Scandinavica,* 81, 164-169.

[23] E, J. and P, O. (1973). Gentamicin in the treatment of sepsis in newborn infants. *Acta Pathologica Microbiologica Scandinavica*, 81, 124-129.

[24] R, S. and P, S. (1973). Clinical experience with gentamicin in neonates. *Acta Pathologica Microbiologica Scandinavica*, 81, 130-136.

[25] R. J., F., et al. (1977). Clindamycin and gentamicin for aerobic and anaerobic sepsis. *Archives of Internal Medicine*, 137, 28-38.

[26] B, F., et al. (1977). Antibiotherapy of Serratia marcescens septicemia in children. *Chemotherapy*, 23, 416-422.

[27] R, M., et al. (2000). A two-step schedule for the treatment of actinomycotic mycetomas. *Acta Dermatovenereologica -Stockholm-*, 80, 378-380.

[28] W, S. and M, E. (1973). Neonatal sepsis due to clostridium perfringens. *Maryland state medical journal*, 22, 61.

[29] M, W., et al. (2006). Treatment of plague with gentamicin or doxycycline in a randomized clinical trial in Tanzania. *Clinical infectious diseases,* 42, 614-621.

[30] I, T. V., et al. (2000). Plague as a biological weapon. *The journal of the American Medical Association*, 283, 2281-2290.

[31] S, H. F. (1957). Ablation therapy in the management of Ménière's disease. *Acta oto-laryngologica*, 132, 1-42.

[32] C-K, R., et al. (2004). Intratympanic Gentamicin for Menière's Disease: a Meta-Analysis. *The Laryngoscope*, 114, 2085-2091.

[33] R, S. D. and O, J. G. (1997). Intratympanic gentamicin for treatment of intractable Meniere's disease: a preliminary report. *The Laryngoscope*, 107, 49-55.

[34] N, J. M., et al. (1992). Chemical labyrinthectomy: local application of gentamicin for the treatment of unilateral Meniere's disease. *Otology and Neurotology,* 13, 18-22.

[35] B, C. and S, C. (1978). 10 Years of experience with intratympanally applied streptomycin (gentamycin) in the therapy of Morbus Menière. *Archives of oto-rhino-laryngology*, 221, 149-152.

[36] O, L. and B, L. and L, A. (1984). Topical gentamycin treatment for disabling Menière's disease. *Acta Oto-Laryngologica* (Stockholm), 412, 74-76.

[37] C, J. (1972). Pathogenesis and treatment of facial paralysis due to malignant external otitis. *The Annals of otology, rhinology, and laryngology,* 81, 648.

[38] Hill, I. and M, M. and B, M. (1980). Successful management of persistent diarrhoea in infants. *South African Medical Journal/Suid-Afrikaanse Mediese Tydskrift*, 58, 241-243.

[39] B, S., et al. (1992). Efficacy of massive dose oral gentamicin therapy in nonbloody persistent diarrhea with associated malnutrition. *Journal of pediatric gastroenterology and nutrition,* 15, 117-124.

[40] B, A. V., et al. (1992). Oral gentamicin is not effective treatment for persistent diarrhea. *Acta paediatrica*, 81, 149-154.

[41] R, R. V. and N, D. L. (1989) Diverticular disease. *Current Problems in Surgery,* 26, 133-189.

[42] H, D. L., et al. (1997). A multicenter study comparing intravenous meropenem with clindamycin plus gentamicin for the treatment of acute gynecologic and obstetric pelvic infections in hospitalized women. *Clinical infectious diseases,* 24, S222-S230.

[43] H, G., et al. (1980). Prospective, randomized comparative study of clindamycin, chloramphenicol, and ticarcillin, each in combination with gentamicin, in therapy for intraabdominal and female genital tract sepsis. *Journal of Infectious Diseases*, 142, 384-393.

[44] W, D. M. and G, R. S. (1990). A randomized comparison of gentamicin-clindamycin and cefoxitin-doxycycline in the treatment of acute pelvic inflammatory disease. *Obstetrics and gynaecology*, 75, 867-872.

[45] M, A. G., et al. (1997). A randomized, prospective study comparing once-daily gentamicin versus thrice-daily gentamicin in the treatment of puerperal infection. *American journal of obstetrics and gynecology*, 177, 786-792.

[46] I, T., et al. (1991). Gentamicin-collagen sponge for local applications: 10 cases of chronic osteomyelitis followed for 1 year. *Acta Orthopaedica*, 62, 592-594.

[47] S, T. S. and S, A. I. and M, S. (1990). Rapid release of gentamicin from collagen sponge. vitro comparison with plastic beads. *Acta Orthopaedica Scandinavica,* 61, 353-356.

[48] W, A. J. and R, B. W. (1979). Management of pulmonary disease in patients with cystic fibrosis. *New England Journal of Medicine*, 335, 179-188.

[49] M, L. I. (1979). Prevention of neurosurgical infection by intraoperative antibiotics. *Neurosurgery*, 5, 339-343.

[50] B, R. S. and C, R. A. (1988). A randomized clinical trial of topical gentamicin after tympanostomy tube placement. *Archives of Otolaryngology—Head and Neck Surgery*, 114, 755-757.

[51] A, (1997). Antimicrobial prophylaxis in surgery. *The Medical Letter*, 39, 97-102.

[52] L, M., et al. (1992). A comparative study of imipenem versus piperacillin plus gentamicin in the initial management of febrile neutropenic patients with haematological malignancies. *Journal of Antimicrobial Chemotherapy,* 30, 843-854.

[53] F, A. G., et al. (2010). Clinical practice guideline for the use of antimicrobial agents in neutropenic patients with cancer: 2010 update by the Infectious Diseases Society of America. *Clinical infectious diseases*, 52, e56-e93.

[54] B, B., et al. (1989). Gentamicin and low dose piperacillin in febrile neutropenic patients. *Journal of Antimicrobial Chemotherapy*, 24, 45-51.

[55] T, R. J., et al. (1999). Once daily ceftriaxone and gentamicin for the treatment of febrile neutropenia. *Archives of disease in childhood*, 80, 125-131.

[56] A, S., et al. (1971). Gentamicin for septicemia in patients with burns. *Journal of Infectious Diseases*, 124, S275-S277.

[57] H, R. P. and M, B. G. and A, W. A. (1970). Topical and systemic antibacterial agents in the treatment of burns. *Annals of surgery*, 172, 370.

[58] M, B. G. (1969). Gentamicin in the management of thermal injuries. *Journal of Infectious Diseases*, 119, 492-503.

[59] Z, D., et al. (1982). Increased burn patient survival with individualized dosages of gentamicin. *Surgery*, 91, 142-149.

[60] Z, D. E., et al. (1991). Initial dosage regimens of gentamicin in patients with burns. *Journal of Burn Care and Research*, 12, 46-50.

[61] F, G. N., et al. (2006). Impact of rapid in situ hybridization testing on coagulase-negative staphylococci positive blood cultures. *Journal of Antimicrobial Chemotherapy,* 58, 154-158.

[62] C, C. H. (2013). Staphylococcus saprophyticus Bacteremia with Pyelonephritis Cured by GM. *Journal of the Formosan Medical Association,* in press

[63] R, D. and R, V. (1999). The body louse as a vector of reemerging human diseases. *Clinical infectious diseases*, 29, 888-911.

[64] S, D. H., et al. (1995). Bartonella (Rochalimaea) quintana bacteremia in inner-city patients with chronic alcoholism. *New England Journal of Medicine,* 332, 424-428.

[65] S, A. and R, D. (1995). Return of trench fever. *Lancet*, 345, 450-451.

[66] F, C., et al. (2002). Bartonella quintana bacteremia among homeless people. *Clinical infectious diseases*, 35, 684-689.

[67] F, C. and R, D. and B, P. (2003). Randomized open trial of gentamicin and doxycycline for eradication of Bartonella quintana from blood in patients with chronic bacteremia. *Antimicrobial agents and chemotherapy*, 47, 2204-2207.

[68] D, A. H. and E, C. E. (1985). Neonatal mortality: effects of selective pediatric interventions. *Pediatrics*, 75, 51-7.

[69] M, E. I. and C, R. W. (2004). Antibiotic regimens for suspected early neonatal sepsis. *Cochrane Database of Systematic Reviews*, 4, CD0044 95.

[70] C, R. H., et al. (2006). Empiric Use of Ampicillin and Cefotaxime, Compared With Ampicillin and Gentamicin, for Neonates at Risk for Sepsis Is Associated With an Increased Risk of Neonatal Death. *Pediatrics*, 117, 67-74.

[71] M, T., et al. (2010). Comparison of ampicillin plus gentamicin vs. penicillin plus gentamicin in empiric treatment of neonates at risk of early onset sepsis. *Acta Paediatrica*, 99, 665-72.

[72] Z, A. K., et al. (2012). Community-based treatment of serious bacterial infections in newborns and young infants: a randomized controlled trial assessing three antibiotic regimens. *The Pediatric Infectious Disease Journal,* 31, 667-72.

[73] N, N., et al. (2013). Effect of Clinical and Histological Chorioamnionitis on the Outcome of Preterm Infants. *American journal of perinatology*, 30,59-68.

[74] G, R. S., et al. (1998). A randomized trial of intrapartum versus immediate postpartum treatment of women with intra-amniotic infection. *Obstetrics and Gynecology*, 72, 823-828.

[75] L, M. E. (1992). New dosing regimens for aminoglycoside antibiotics. *Annals of internal medicine*, 117, 693-694.

[76] L, D. J., et al. (2010). Daily Compared With 8-Hour Gentamicin for the Treatment of Intrapartum Chorioamnionitis: A Randomized Controlled Trial. *Obstetrics and Gynecology*, 115, 344-349.

[77] O, R. J. (2004). Reducing the risk of postoperative endophthalmitis. *Survey of ophthalmology*, 49, S55.

[78] L, O. J., et al. (1997). Association between nonadministration of subconjunctival cefuroxime and postoperative endophthalmitis. *Journal of cataract and refractive surgery*, 23, 889.

[79] M, P. G., et al. (2002). Prophylactic intracameral cefuroxime: efficacy in preventing endophthalmitis after cataract surgery. *Journal of cataract and refractive surgery*, 28, 977-981.

[80] A, M. S. and A, M. A. (2010). Use of povidone-iodine drop instead of sub-conjunctival injection of dexamethasone and gentamicin combination at the end of phacoemulsification cataract surgery. *Mymensingh Medical Journal*, 19, 232-5.

[81] F, H. W., et al. (2004). Current management of endophthalmitis. *International ophthalmology clinics*, 44, 115-137.

[82] L, N. A. (1996). Microbiologic factors and visual outcome in the endophthalmitis vitrectomy study. *American Journal of Ophthalmology*, 122, 830-46.

[83] L, G. A., et al. (2008). Acute-Onset Endophthalmitis after Clear Corneal Cataract Surgery (1996–2005). *Ophthalmology*, 115, 473-476.

[84] G, J. P. (1991). Filters and Antibiotics in Irrigating Solution for Cataract Surgery. *Journal of cataract and refractive surgery*, 17, 385.

[85] B, J. L. and B, G. D. (2006). Prospective randomized controlled trial of the effect of intracameral vancomycin and gentamicin on macular retinal thickness and visual function following cataract surgery. *Journal of cataract and refractive surgery,* 32, 789-794.

[86] C, G. and F, X. and L, J. (2012). The effects of aminoglycoside antibiotics on platelet aggregation and blood coagulation. *Clinical and Applied Thrombosis/Hemostasis*, 18, 538-541.

[87] R, S. D., (2010). Clinical hints and precipitating factors in patients suffering from Meniere's disease. *Otolaryngologic clinics of North America,* 43, 1011-1017.

[88] N, J. M., et al. (1993). Intratympanic gentamicin instillation as treatment of unilateral Meniere's disease: update of an ongoing study. *Otology and Neurotology*, 14, 278-282.

[89] K, D. M., et al. (2000). Intratympanic gentamicin for the treatment of unilateral Meniere's disease. *The Laryngoscope*, 110, 1298-1305.

[90] S, L., et al. (2001). Intratympanic dexamethasone, intratympanic gentamicin, and endolymphatic sac surgery for intractable vertigo in Meniere's disease. *Otolaryngology--Head and Neck Surgery*, 125, 537-543.

[91] R, M. J. (1999). Immunologic aspects of Meniere's disease. *American journal of otolaryngology,* 20, 161-165.

[92] H, C., et al. (2010). Transtympanic steroids for Meniere's disease. *Otology and Neurotology*, 31, 162-167.

[93] D, K. M. and S, A. (2004). Intratympanic steroid perfusion for the treatment of Meniere's disease: a retrospective study. *Ear, nose, and throat journal*, 83, 394-398.

[94] C, A., et al. (2005). Transtympanic gentamicin and fibrin tissue adhesive for treatment of unilateral Meniere's disease: effects on vestibular function. *Otolaryngology-Head and Neck Surgery*, 133, 929-935.

[95] C, A. P., et al. (2012). Intratympanic Treatment of Intractable Unilateral Ménière Disease Gentamicin or Dexamethasone? A Randomized Controlled Trial. *Otolaryngology--Head and Neck Surgery*, 146, 430-437.

[96] H, L. C., et al. (2009). High-dose intratympanic gentamicin instillations for treatment of Meniere's disease: long-term results. *Acta Otolaryngologica*, 129, 1420-1424.

[97] D, L. P. and P, P. A. (2011). Intratympanic gentamicin in Ménière's disease: our experience. *Journal of Laryngology and Otology*, 125, 363-369.

[98] P, R. J., et al. (2008). Intratympanic gentamicin therapy for control of vertigo in unilateral Ménière's disease: a prospective, double-blind, randomized, placebo-controlled trial. *Acta Oto-laryngologica*, 128, 876-880.

[99] P, N. and R, L. J. (2005). Vestibular function at the end of intratympanic gentamicin treatment of patients with Ménière's disease. *Journal of Vestibular Research*, 15, 49-58.

[100] S, R. and K, H. (2004). Selective vestibular ablation by intratympanic gentamicin in patients with unilateral active Ménière's disease: a prospective, double-blind, placebo-controlled, randomized clinical trial. *Acta Oto-laryngologica*, 124, 172-175.

[101] V, P., et al. (1998). Vestibular compensation revisited. *Otolaryngology--Head and Neck Surgery*, 119, 34-42.

[102] M, M., et al. (2007). Preoperative vestibular ablation with gentamicin and vestibular 'prehab' enhance postoperative recovery after surgery for pontine angle tumours--first report. *Acta Oto-Laryngologica*, 127, 1236-1240.

[103] T, F., et al. (2009). Vestibular PREHAB and gentamicin before schwannoma surgery may improve long-term postural function. Journal of Neurology, *Neurosurgery and Psychiatry*, 80, 1254-1260.

[104] R, J., et al. (2012). Effect of Peritoneal Lavage with Clindamycin-Gentamicin Solution on Infections after Elective Colorectal Cancer Surgery. *Journal of the American College of Surgeons*, 214, 202-207.

[105] W, J. L., et al. (2011). Safety and efficacy of once-daily nasal irrigation for the treatment of pediatric chronic rhinosinusitis. *The Laryngoscope*, 121, 1989-2000.

[106] H, T. C., et al. (1992). CDC definitions of nosocomial surgical site infections, 1992: a modification of CDC definitions of surgical wound infections. *Infection Control and Hospital Epidemiology*, 13, 606-608.

[107] S, R. J., et al. (1992). Consensus paper on the surveillance of surgical wound infections. *American Journal of Infection Control*, 20, 263-270.

[108] B, E., et al. (2010). Gentamicin-collagen sponge for infection prophylaxis in colorectal surgery. *New England Journal of Medicine*, 363, 1038-1049.

[109] F, Ö., et al. (2003). Antibiotic concentrations in serum and wound fluid after local gentamicin or intravenous dicloxacillin prophylaxis in cardiac surgery. *Scandinavian journal of infectious diseases*, 35, 251-254.

[110] R, Z. and F, W. (2003). Collagen as a carrier for on-site delivery of antibacterial drugs. *Advanced drug delivery reviews*, 55, 1679-1698.

[111] R, H. and N, P. (1997). Prevention of wound infection in elective colorectal surgery by local application of a gentamicin-containing collagen sponge. *The European journal of surgery. Acta chirurgica*. 578, 31-35.

[112] G, G. G. V., et al. (1999). Effectiveness of collagen–gentamicin implant for treatment of "dirty" abdominal wounds. *World journal of surgery*, 23, 123-127.

[113] N, M. P., et al. (2005). Prospective, randomized trial examining the role of gentamycin-containing collagen sponge in the reduction of postoperative morbidity in rectal cancer patients: early results and surprising outcome at 3-year follow-up. *International journal of colorectal disease*, 20, 114-120.

[114] Y, I., et al. (2010). Effect of gentamicin-absorbed collagen in wound healing in pilonidal sinus surgery: a prospective randomized study. *Journal of International Medical Research*, 38, 1029-1033.

[115] A, R. E., et al. (2010). Local Administration of Antibiotics by Gentamicin–Collagen Sponge does not Improve Wound Healing or Reduce Recurrence Rate After Pilonidal Excision with Primary Suture: A Prospective Randomized Controlled Trial. *World journal of surgery*, 34, 3042-3048.

[116] H, B., et al. (2003). Efficacy and tolerance of a new gentamicin collagen fleece (Septocoll®) after surgical treatment of a pilonidal sinus. *Colorectal Disease*, 5 222-227.

[117] F, Ö., et al. (2006). Cost effectiveness of local collagen-gentamicin as prophylaxis for sternal wound infections in different risk groups. *Scandinavian Cardiovascular Journal*, 40, 117-125.

[118] M, W. J. and S, P. and T, R. L. (2008). Sternal wound infections. *Best practice and research clinical anaesthesiology*, 22, 423-436.

[119] T, G. H., et al. (2004). Prevention and management of deep sternal wound infection. *Semin. Thorac. Cardiovasc. Surg.*,16,62–69

[120] S, C., et al. (2012). Gentamicin-collagen sponge reduces sternal wound complications after heart surgery: a controlled, prospectively randomized, double-blind study. *The Journal of Thoracic and Cardiovascular Surgery*, 143, 194-200.

[121] B, E., et al. (2010). Effect of an implantable gentamicin-collagen sponge on sternal wound infections following cardiac surgery. *The journal of the American Medical Association*, 304, 755-762.

[122] F, Ö., (2007). Local collagen-gentamicin for prevention of sternal wound infections: the LOGIP trial. *Apmis*, 115, 1016-1021.

[123] E, A. and V, M. and W, K. (2005). Prophylaxis of sternal wound infections with gentamicin-collagen implant: randomized controlled study in cardiac surgery. *The Journal of hospital infection*, 59, 108-112.

[124] J, G. and H, M. and N, N. (1996). Hidradenitis suppurativa-characteristics and consequences. *Clinical and experimental dermatology,* 21, 419-423.

[125] B, T. J. and R, T. and O, I. F. (1998). Hidradenitis suppurativa. *Southern medical journal,* 91, 1107-1114.

[126] J, G. B. and W, P. (1998). Topical clindamycin versus systemic tetracycline in the treatment of hidradenitis suppurativa. *Journal of the American Academy of Dermatology,* 39, 971-974.

[127] B, M. G., et al. (2008). Surgical Treatment of Hidradenitis Suppurativa with Gentamicin Sulfate: A Prospective Randomized Study. *Dermatologic Surgery*, 34, 224-227.

[128] L, B. A., et al. (2012). Topical Application of a Gentamicin-Collagen Sponge Combined with Systemic Antibiotic Therapy for the Treatment of Diabetic Foot Infections of Moderate Severity A Randomized, Controlled, Multicenter Clinical Trial. *Journal of the American Podiatric Medical Association*, 102, 223-232.

[129] P, D. (1992). Human leishmaniases: epidemiology and public health aspects. *World Health Statistics Quarterly*, 45, 267-275.

[130] M, A. J. (2005). Cutaneous leishmaniasis in the returning traveler. *Infectious disease clinics of North America*, 19, 241-266.

[131] B, A., et al. (2013). Topical Paromomycin with or without Gentamicin for Cutaneous Leishmaniasis. *New England Journal of Medicine*, 368, 524-532.

[132] A, D. and T, P. and R.A.P.D. Group. (2012). Do topical antibiotics reduce exit site infection rates and peritonitis episodes in peritoneal dialysis patients? The Pan Thames Renal Audit. *Journal of Nephrology*, 25, 819-824.

[133] S, T. (1993). The economic impact of infected total joint arthroplasty. *Instructional course lectures*, 42, 349.

[134] Z, W. and O, P. Management of infection associated with prosthetic joints. *Infection*, 31, 99-108.

[135] K, C. J., et al. (1997). Incidence and sources of native and prosthetic joint infection: a community based prospective survey. *Annals of the rheumatic diseases,* 56, 470-475.

[136] H, P. H., et al. (2004). Two-stage revision hip arthroplasty for infection: comparison between the interim use of antibiotic-loaded cement beads and a spacer prosthesis. *The Journal of Bone and Joint Surgery*, 86, 1989-1997.

[137] T, P., et al. (1999). Prosthetic joint infection: when can prosthesis salvage be considered? *Clinical infectious diseases*, 29, 292-295.

[138] M, D. J. and F, R. and I, D. (1989). Two-stage reconstruction of a total hip arthroplasty because of infection. *Journal of bone and joint surgery*. 71, 828-834.

[139] L, L., et al. (2006). Treatment of bone and joint infections caused by Gram-negative bacilli with a cefepime–fluoroquinolone combination. *Clinical Microbiology and Infection*, 12, 1030-1033.

[140] S, D. J. and W, R. (1978). Gram negative bone and joint infection: sixty patients treated with amikacin. *Clinical Orthopaedics and Related Research,* 134, 268-274.

[141] S, E., et al. (2003). The infected total hip arthroplasty. *Instructional course lectures,* 52, 223.

[142] K, K. H., et al. (2001). Impregnation of vancomycin, gentamicin, and cefotaxime in a cement spacer for two-stage cementless reconstruction in infected total hip arthroplasty. *The Journal of arthroplasty*, 16, 882-892.

[143] Y, K., et al. (2009). Cement spacer loaded with antibiotics for infected implants of the hip joint. *The Journal of arthroplasty*, 24, 83.

[144] Y, A., et al. (1997). The outcome of two-stage arthroplasty using a custom-made interval spacer to treat the infected hip. *The Journal of arthroplasty*, 12, 615-623.

[145] L, J. R., et al. (1994). Treatment of the infected total hip arthroplasty with a two-stage reimplantation protocol. *Clinical orthopaedics and related research,* 301, 205-212.

[146] S, B. D., et al. (2004). Systemic Safety of High-Dose Antibiotic-Loaded Cement Spacers after Resection of an Infected Total Knee Arthroplasty. *Clinical Orthopaedics and Related Research*, 427, 47-51.

[147] M, M. P., et al. (2011). A randomized controlled trial of nebulized gentamicin in non–cystic fibrosis bronchiectasis. *American journal of respiratory and critical care medicine,* 183, 491-499.

[148] K, S., et al. (2009). Success of an infection control program to reduce the spread of carbapenem-resistant Klebsiella pneumoniae. *Infection Control and Hospital Epidemiology*, 30, 447-452.

[159] C.f.D.C.a.P. (2009). Guidance for control of infections with carbapenem-resistant or carbapenemase-producing Enterobacteriaceae in acute care facilities. *Morbidity and Mortality Weekly Report*, 58, 256-260.

[150] L, S. O., et al. (2012). A randomized, double-blind, placebo-controlled trial of selective digestive decontamination using oral gentamicin and oral polymyxin E for eradication of carbapenem-resistant Klebsiella pneumoniae carriage. *Infection Control and Hospital Epidemiology*, 33, 14-19.

[151] Y, E. J. (1995). An overview of human brucellosis. *Clinical infectious diseases,* 21, 283-289.

[152] C, J., et al. (1996). Complications associated with Brucella melitensis infection: a study of 530 cases. *Medicine*, 75, 195-211.

[153] R, M. R. H., et al. (2006). Efficacy of gentamicin plus doxycycline versus streptomycin plus doxycycline in the treatment of brucellosis in humans. *Clinical infectious diseases*, 42, 1075-1080.

[154] S, J., et al. (2004). A randomized, double-blind study to assess the optimal duration of doxycycline treatment for human brucellosis. *Clinical infectious diseases*, 39, 1776-1782.

[155] S, J., et al. (1997). Treatment of human brucellosis with doxycycline and gentamicin. *Antimicrobial agents and chemotherapy*, 41, 80-84.

[156] D, D. T., et al. (1999). Plague manual: epidemiology, distribution, surveillance and control/principal authors: David T. Dennis, Kenneth L.

Gage, Norman G. Gratz, Jack D. Poland, Evgueni Tikhomirov, World Health Organization. Epidemic Disease Control.

[157] K, J. L. and W, R. A. (2005). Risk of person-to-person transmission of pneumonic plague. *Clinical Infectious Diseases*, 40, 1166-1172.

[158] W, J. D., et al. (2000). Susceptibilities of Yersinia pestis strains to 12 antimicrobial agents. *Antimicrobial agents and chemotherapy*, 44, 1995-1996.

[159] B, W. R., et al. (1998). Antibiotic treatment of experimental pneumonic plague in mice. *Antimicrobial agents and chemotherapy*, 42, 675-681.

[160] L, M., et al. (1989). A multicenter therapeutic study of 1100 children with brucellosis. *The Pediatric infectious disease journal*, 8, 75-78.

[161] R, M. H., et al. (2010). Comparison of the efficacy of gentamicin for 5 days plus doxycycline for 8 weeks versus streptomycin for 2 weeks plus doxycycline for 45 days in the treatment of human brucellosis: a randomized clinical trial. *Journal of Antimicrobial Chemotherapy*, 65, 1028-1035.

[162] B, L. L., et al. (2004). Gentamicin and tetracyclines for the treatment of human plague: review of 75 cases in New Mexico, 1985–1999. *Clinical infectious diseases,* 38, 663-669.

Reviewed by Dr. BinBin Wu.

Reviewer' affiliation: Department of Internal Medicine, Changhua Christian Hospital, Taiwan

In: Gentamicin
Editor: Emilie Kruger

ISBN: 978-1-62808-841-0
© 2013 Nova Science Publishers, Inc.

Chapter 2

GENTAMICIN AND PARTICLE ENGINEERING: FROM AN OLD MOLECULE TO INNOVATIVE DRUG DELIVERY SYSTEMS

Giulia Auriemma, Mariateresa Stigliani, Paola Russo,
*Pasquale Del Gaudio and Rita P. Aquino**
Department of Pharmacy, University of Salerno, Fisciano, Italy

ABSTRACT

Gentamicin sulfate (GS) is one of the most important antibiotics of the family "Aminoglycosides" worldwide used for its effective bactericidal activities, low bacterial resistance and post-antibiotic effects, and moderate cost. GS, similarly to other members of the "aminoglycosides" family, shows low effectiveness when administered orally, therefore, the antibiotic is usually administered intravenously or intramuscularly. However, due to its pharmacokinetics and biopharmaceutical properties, multiple systemic daily administrations are needed to achieve good antibiotic concentrations; this may cause serious side effects such as ototoxicity and nephrotoxicity which limit its clinical exploitation.

A local administration which can deliver high dose of drug directly to the site of infection, while minimizing systemic exposure, can overcome these limits. In this case, appropriate dosage forms must be

* Corresponding author, aquinorp@unisa.it.

designed to obtain a local controlled drug release and to solve biopharmaceutical and pharmacokinetic issues that hinder the optimal use of GS in the clinical practice.

In the last few years microtechnologies have been applied as tool to innovate GS delivery. The major drawback encountered when formulating GS microparticles is its high hygroscopicity. In fact, as it is well known, hygroscopicity may modulate the moisture content of microparticles in the final dosage form and it is correlated to chemical or physical instability and poor flowability of the final powder product.

The present chapter briefly describes the critical properties of gentamicin from both a pharmacological and technological point of view.

Particularly, the aim of the chapter is to illustrates "particle engineering" strategies, i.e. spray drying and supercritical fluid techniques, adopted to improve technological properties of GS raw material. A special focus will be on i) the development of dry powders for inhalation, ii) the development of microparticulate powder for topical application in wound care. Both approaches allow to obtain micronized gentamicin powders, easy to handle, stable for long time and suitable for pulmonary and topical administration, respectively.

Keywords: Gentamicin; Particle Engineering; Spray Drying; Dry Powder Inhalers; Cystic Fibrosis; Supercritical Assisted Atomization; Wound bacterial infections

1. INTRODUCTION

Gentamicin sulfate (GS) is an aminoglycoside antibiotic worldwide used for the treatment of severe infections caused by both Gram-positive and, especially, Gram-negative bacteria (Forge and Schacht 2000). The "Amynoglycosides" family includes other active compounds with the same basic chemical structure, such as amikacin, arbekacin, kanamycin, neomycin, netilmicin, paromomycin, streptomycin, rhodostreptomycin, vancomycin, apramycin and tobramycin. Aminoglycosides are very effective bactericidal antibiotics that inhibit protein synthesis (Abdelghany, Quinn et al. 2012) and damage the plasma membrane (Davis 1987) binding to the 30S ribosomal subunit of bacterial cells. GS is one of the most commonly used for its low cost and reliable activity against gram-negative aerobes. This antibiotic exhibits rapid concentration-dependent killing action: increasing concentrations with higher dosages increases both the rate and the extent of bacterial cell death. In addition, GS presents significant post antibiotic effects demonstrating a persistent suppression of bacterial growth also after short exposure (Gonzalez and Spencer 1998). Like other aminoglycosides, GS shows low effectiveness when administered orally because it is poorly absorbed from the gastrointestinal tract (Balmayor, Baran et al. 2012). Therefore, gentamicin is usually administered intravenously or intramuscularly. However, due to its biopharmaceutical and pharmacokinetics properties (e.g. limited permeability through endothelial cell membranes and short half-life) (Haswani, Nettey et al. 2006; Abdelghany, Quinn et al. 2012), high doses and multiple systemic daily administrations are needed to ensure adequate therapeutic serum concentrations; this may cause serious side effects such as ototoxicity and nephrotoxicity which strongly limit its therapeutic use (Ito, Kusawake et al. 2005; Selimoglu 2007; Balakumar, Rohilla et al. 2010). These problems can be overcome by local administration which can deliver high dose of drug directly to the site of infection, while minimizing systemic exposure (de Jesús Valle, López et al. 2007; Krasko, Golenser et al. 2007).

In the past, the conventional approach when dealing with such substances was to modify their chemical structure. Indeed, in the last few years there is a continuous research in the development of processes and techniques that allow to transform active pharmaceutical ingredients (APIs) into new dosage forms providing a solution to the above mentioned problems (Buttini, Colombo et al. 2012).

In fact, the so-called "new drug delivery systems" are able to modify biopharmaceutical and pharmacokinetic properties of the API, to control its release rate, and to obtain a site specific delivery, reducing side effects. All these aspects may increase both the therapeutic efficacy and the safety of known drugs allowing an optimal use in clinical practice (Tiwari, R. et al. 2012).

The design of a controlled drug delivery system requires simultaneous consideration of several factors, such as API properties, route of administration, nature of delivery vehicle, mechanism of drug release, ability of targeting, and biocompatibility (Figure 1), but it is not easy to achieve all these in one system (Coelho, Ferreira et al. 2010). Moreover, reliability and reproducibility of any drug delivery system is the most important factor while designing such a system.

All efforts to enhance therapeutic value of both new and old drugs have been the key driver in particle engineering, a term used to describe particle generation techniques driven by rational design of particle size, morphology and chemical composition (Mack, Horvath et al. 2012). Today, the particle is no longer seen as a passive carrier, but rather as an essential part of the drug delivery system (Vehring 2008).

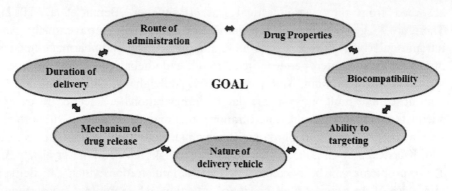

Paolino, Sinha et al. 2006.

Figure 1. Design requirement for a drug delivery systems.

The main goal of particle engineering is to incorporate desirable attributes, such as narrow particle-size distribution, improved dispersibility, enhanced drug stability, optimized bioavailability, sustained release and/or precise targeting, into particle while taking into account the specifics of formulation design and drug delivery requirements (Chow, Tong et al. 2007).

This chapter provides a review of two different "particle engineering" strategies, with special focus on spray drying and supercritical fluid technologies, with the aim to develop gentamicin based microparticles for pulmonary administration in cystic fibrosis (CF) or for topical application in wound care.

2. PHARMACEUTICAL PARTICLE ENGINEERING

The key for successfully developing and manufacturing a new dosage form is the study of the relationship between particles properties and final product performance.

Particle shape, size, adhesiveness, morphology, roughness are some of the properties that are usually evaluated. However, investigation on wettability, density, surface chemistry, plasticity, hardness, brittleness, moisture adsorption capability, permeability, and a tendency to gain electrostatic charge are necessary to determine the performance of the final product (Parikh 2011).

Among these, particle size distribution and particle shape usually constitute the critical variables of a pharmaceutical manufacturing process, and also affect quality attributes, such as:

- flow and packing properties, mixing and segregation of powders, rheological characteristics of liquid and semisolid formulations;
- content and dose uniformity and other properties related to the physicochemical stability;
- dissolution rate and bioavailability of APIs;
- drug release rate for sustained and controlled release formulations;
- aerosolization behavior and the corresponding performance of respiratory formulations;
- in-vivo particle distribution and deposition, absorption rate and clearance time (especially for aerosols and different colloidal systems designed for targeted drug delivery) (Parikh 2011).

The possibility to design tailor made particles by "particles engineering" allows to well control and optimize technological and biopharmaceutical properties in order to obtain the desired results.

Particles engineering approaches range from traditional micronization methods to novel and sophisticated Micro- or Nano-encapsulation techniques.

As well known, traditional methods used to produce micrometric particles, such as crushing/milling and crystallization/precipitation, lead to products with a poor control of particle size, shape and morphology (Chow, Tong et al. 2007; Hu, Zhao et al. 2008; Joshi 2011).

Spray drying (SD) and supercritical fluid (SCF) technologies represent new and interesting routes for particle formation, which avoids most of the drawbacks of the traditional processes.

2.1. Spray Drying

Spray drying is a one-step, continuous and scalable drying process which converts liquid feeds (i.e., solutions, suspensions and emulsions) into dry powders. During this process, the liquid feed is first atomized to a spray form (atomization step) that is put immediately into thermal contact with a hot gas, resulting in the rapid evaporation of the droplets (drying step). The dried particles are then separated from the heated gas by means of a cyclone (separation step) (Pilcer and Amighi 2010).

In the last few years, this technique is gaining more and more attention as approach to form engineered API particles with characteristics that cannot be readily achieved using other manufacturing techniques (Sou, Meeusen et al. 2011). The chemical composition of the solid particulates depends on the content within the feed solution, whereas particle size and morphology are strongly dependent on process parameters such as liquid and gas feed rate, inlet temperature, gas pressure and aspiration (Vehring 2008; Maas, Schaldach et al. 2011). Actually, spray drying is the most commonly used technique to generate inhalable engineered particles (Parlati, Colombo et al. 2009; Wu, Hayes et al. 2013).

2.1.1. Spray Drying And Pulmonary Delivery

Inhalation therapy, highly recommended in pathologies affecting the lung (i.e. asthma, cystic fibrosis, chronic obstructive pulmonary disease), consists of drug administration directly to the lung in form of micronized droplets or solid microparticles, reducing the overall required dose and decreasing systemic exposure to the drug and formulation excipients (Labiris and Dolovich 2003).

The possibility to deliver high doses, the greater stability compared to liquid formulations and the problems of pressurized metered dose inhaler (pMDI) use have recently led research in the direction of formulating dry powder inhalers (DPIs) (Islam; Son and McConville 2008). DPIs is particularly challenging since the preparation of a "respirable" formulation and the selection of an adequate device for metering and aerosolizing the dose are both required. Therefore, formulation and device for inhalation have to be developed together (Friebel, Steckel et al. 2012).

Currently there are essentially four types of DPIs (Islam):

- Single-unit dose (capsule); This inhaler requires the patient to load a single hard gelatin capsule containing the powder formulation into the device before each use. This is a very common type of DPI device currently available on market.
- Single-unit dose (disposable); It is a device containing a pre-metered amount of a single dose that is discarded after use.
- Multi-unit dose (pre-metered unit replaceable set); Multi-unit devices deliver individual doses from pre-metered replaceable blisters, disks, dimples or tubes.

- Multiple dose (reservoir); Multiple dose reservoir inhalers contain a bulk amount of drug powder in the device with a built in mechanism to meter a single dose from the bulk and individual doses are delivered with each actuation.

It is very difficult to compare the performances of different DPIs (which have different design, resistance, mechanism of drug dispersion) without investigating their performances using the same drug formulation and same inspiratory force in a controlled environment. There is no comprehensive information (or data with limited information/access) on the comparative studies based on the performance of various devices. Therefore, it is extremely difficult to make a straightforward comparison on the performances of various devices (Islam). The only certainty is that the effective delivery of drugs from inhaler devices depends not only on the design of the device but also on the drug dry powder formulation.

The biggest issue encountered when formulating a dry powder for inhalation is to guarantee the aerosolization and the deposition at the appropriate site of the respiratory tract. A failure in deposition may result in a failure of efficacy. The aerodynamic behavior of inhaled particles depends on the so-called "aerodynamic diameter" (Dae), a spherical equivalent diameter that derives from the equivalence between the inhaled particle and a sphere of unit density (ρ_0) undergoing sedimentation at the same rate (Eq. 1).

$$Dae = Dv \sqrt{\frac{\rho}{\chi \rho_0}} \qquad (1)$$

where Dv is the volume-equivalent diameter, ρ is the particle density and χ is the shape factor (Depreter, Pilcer et al. 2013). Hence, particle geometry, density and volume diameter are the main characteristics to customize since they affect dry powder inhalation performance (Buttini, Colombo et al. 2012). It is generally accepted that particles with an aerodynamic diameter of 1-5 μm (referred to as the "respirable range") tend to deposit in the lungs, while particles larger than 5 μm are trapped in the upper respiratory tract. However, owing to their small size, microparticles are extremely adhesive and cohesive resulting in low dispersibility and, consequently, poor flow properties (Chew and Chan 2002). One way to improve the aerodynamic performance of a spray-dried powder is through the addition of excipients (Shoyele, Sivadas et al. 2011). Many compounds that could enhance drug delivery outcomes also have the potential to irritate or injure the lungs, so when formulating an inhalation dosage form the structural and functional integrity of respiratory epithelium must be respected (Telko and Hickey 2005). The current excipients approved by the Food and Drug Administration (FDA) for respiratory drug delivery are very limited in number and not accepted world-wide. The array of potential excipients is limited to compounds that are biocompatible to the lung and can easily be metabolized or cleared, like sugars (lactose, mannitol and glucose) and hydrophobic additives (magnesium stearate, DSPC). In the last few years, amino acids (AAs) have been tested as alternative excipients due to their ability to decrease hygroscopicity and improve surface activity and charge density of particles. Different studies have demonstrated that co-spray-drying of few selected amino acids with active compounds provides enhanced aerodynamic properties of the final dry powders (Li, Seville et al. 2005; Seville, Learoyd et al. 2007).

Moreover, as amino acids are endogenous substances, they might not present a major risk of toxicity to the lungs (Pilcer and Amighi 2010). Different amino acids such as arginine, aspartic acid, phenylalanine, threonine and leucine have been tested in dry powder formulations as enhancer of aerodynamic properties, the most noteworthy effects have been observed with leucine (Depreter, Pilcer et al. 2013). For example, selection of appropriate solvent systems and leucine concentration has allowed to produce highly respirable β-oestradiol spray-dried powders (Rabbani and Seville 2005). The influence of leucine amount on powder dispersibility and manufacturability has been reported. A 10–20% (w/w) of leucine in spray-dried ethanol or water solutions gives good aerosolization characteristics to peptides or sodium cromoglycate (Chew, Shekunov et al. 2005; Rabbani and Seville 2005; Padhi, Chougule et al. 2006). It is suggested that addition of leucine results in less cohesive particles and in a decrease of particle size due to the surfactant behavior of leucine, reducing the size of droplets produced during atomization (Vehring 2008). Spray-dried isoleucine has also been shown to improve the aerosol performance and stability of various formulations. Trileucine has also been proven to be an efficient surface active agent able to produce corrugated particles of low cohesivity (Lechuga-Ballesteros, Charan et al. 2008). In this case, the stabilization mechanism seems to be different: as a result of its surface activity, trileucine molecules can orient the hydrophobic groups towards the air at the air/liquid interface during the drying process, providing a hydrophobic surface to the dry particle, thereby contributing to the observed improved aerosol efficiency.

2.1.2. Novel gentamicin DPI (Dry Powder Inhaler) for Cystic Fibrosis Treatment

The aim of our research was to develop inhalable GS powders with satisfying aerodynamic properties and good stability profile by spray drying for the treatment of lung infections in cystic fibrosis (CF). This is the most common lethal genetically inherited disease of the Western World (Shur, Nevell et al. 2008). Pulmonary infections are the major cause of morbidity and mortality in CF, with *Pseudomonas aeruginosa* (Pa) acting as the principal pathogen. The viscous mucus lining the lung of CF patients impairs the mucociliary function, facilitating recurrent and chronic respiratory infections caused mainly by Pa but also by *Haemophilus influenza* and *Bulkolderia cepacia* (Mukhopadhyay, Singh et al. 1996; Ramsey, Pepe et al. 1999).

Treatment of lung disease by antibiotics is an accepted standard in cystic fibrosis cure aimed to reduce decline in lung function and number of hospitalizations (Prayle and Smyth 2010). Various clinical studies on GS inhalation treatment in CF patients chronically infected with Pa have shown that antibiotic solutions for aerosol treatment produce both subjective and objective improvement (Mugabe, Azghani et al. 2005; Abdelghany, Quinn et al. 2012). Interestingly, among aminoglycosides, GS has shown the ability to partially restore the expression of the functional protein CFTR (cystic fibrosis transmembrane conductance regulator) in CF mouse models bearing class I nonsense mutations (Wilschanski, Famini et al. 2000; Clancy, Bebok et al. 2001; Du, Jones et al. 2002; Wilschanski, Yahav et al. 2003). In particular, Du and coll. (Du, Jones et al. 2002) demonstrated that GS was able to induce the expression of a higher CFTR level compared to tobramycin.

Regarding the use of gentamicin sulfate in the treatment of airways infections and class I CFTR mutations, the main problem is its reduced penetration in the endobronchial space after intravenous administration, combined with its high systemic toxicity. Since GS peak sputum concentrations are only 12 to 20% of the peak serum concentrations (Mendelman, Smith et al. 1985) to achieve adequate drug concentrations at the site of action, it is necessary to use large intravenous doses, which may produce serum levels associated with renal and oto-toxicity. These problems can be overcome by the use of aerosolized GS, which can deliver high dose of drug directly to the lungs, while minimizing systemic exposure.

The major drawback encountered when formulating GS microparticles is its high hydrophilia. As its high hydrophilia guarantees a rapid drug solubility and diffusion in the fluids lining the lung, as it may cause high hygroscopicity and instability, preventing the formulation of a stable and respirable dry powder.

In order to reduce hygroscopicity and to increase powder dispersibility and stability, GS was spray dried alone or with leucine (Leu) as flowability enhancer at different concentrations from water or various hydro-alcoholic solutions (Aquino, Prota et al. 2012).

As reported in Table 1, addition of the organic co-solvent (isopropanol-ISO) into the water feed was extremely helpful in terms of process yield. Differently, Leu addition did not have a linear effect on spray drying yield, especially in hydro-alcoholic solutions.

Table 1. Physical characteristics of spray dried particles: liquid feeds composition, process yield, particle size and bulk density

Sample code	Water/ISO (%v/v)	Leu content (%w/w)	Process yield (%)	d_{50} (μm) and span	Bulk density (g/ml)
G	100% H_2O	0	53.9±1.0	4.06 (1.63)	0.07±0.02
GISO3	7/3	0	85.5±0.7	4.24 (1.97)	0.19±0.02
GISO3-Leu15	7/3	15	82.0±2.1	3.90 (1.62)	0.34±0.01

Optimized process parameters led to micronized powders with d_{50} similar for all batches produced (Table 1), with no evident effect of solvent and Leu content on the particles diameter.

Organic co-solvent and Leu had a massive effect on hygroscopicity, too. In particular, by adding 30% v/v of ISO into the aqueous feed, humidity uptake by GS powders was reduced from 10.5% (water) to 4.8% (water/ISO) after exposure at room conditions. These effects may be explained by the addition of the lower-soluble component (Leu) into the liquid feeds, able to reach the critical concentration for shell formation as the droplet evaporation progresses during spray-drying process (Vehring 2008). Such enrichment in Leu at the particle surface seems to slow down water uptake of hygroscopic drug such as GS and, potentially, increase powder flowability (Shur, Nevell et al. 2008).

Leu effect on spray-dried powders appears clearly, after microscopy studies, as an evident increase in particle corrugation. As an example, SEM pictures of particles dried from 7/3 water/ISO ratio solutions were reported in Figure 2.

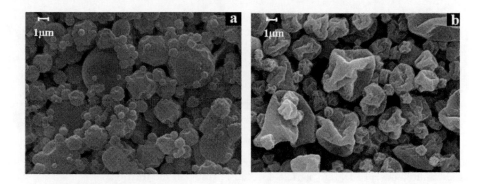

Figure 2. SEM pictures of powders dried from water/IPA 7/3 v/v systems containing: a) GISO3; b) GISO3-Leu15.

As well known, the morphology of spray-dried particles is strongly influenced by the solubility of the components and their initial saturation in the liquid feeds. GS, freely soluble in water, led to the formation of spherical and smooth particles when spray dried alone (Figure 2). According to previous observations (Lechuga-Ballesteros, Charan et al. 2008; Boraey, Hoe et al. 2013), during the co-spray drying process, the saturation of the lower-soluble component (Leu) may increase faster than that of hydrophilic one (GS), due to the preferential evaporation of alcohol and the associated change in the solvent/co-solvent ratio. This led to the formation of a primary solid shell which collapsed, hence corrugated microparticles were formed. As the relative amount of the less soluble component increased, particle corrugation was more and more evident; particles from almost spherical became raisins like or irregularly wrinkled.

By modifying particle shape and corrugation degree, Leu influenced powder bulk density too. In fact, powders processed from hydro-alcoholic systems showed lower bulk density values than those spray-dried from water, whereas Leu inclusion up to 15% (w/w) led to higher density powders (Table 1). As well known, differences in bulk density influence the amount of powder chargeable into the capsules for the inhalation, which shifted from 60 mg for neat GS to 120 mg for GS/15% Leu. The possibility to charge higher amount of drug into the device allows to reduce the number of actuations required, enhancing patient's compliance.

Table 2. Aerodynamic properties of spray-dried powders after single stage glass impinger deposition experiments; device TURBOSPIN, charged with capsules type 2 (mean ± SD of three experiments)

Sample code	ED (%)	FPD (mg)	FPF (%)
G	/	/	/
GISO3	90.9±7.9	7.5±4.9	13.4±8.5
GISO3-Leu15	99.1±0.3	50.4±0.8	49.4±0.8

ED, emitted dose; FPD, fine particle dose; FPF, fine particle fraction.

As aerodynamic properties, it is important to note that neat GS dried from water (G) was a cohesive and sticky material, unable to be aerosolized. Indeed, GS spray drying from hydroalcoholic solvent (e.g. GISO3) reduced powder cohesivity and enabled the aerosolization process; however, the resulting aerodynamic properties were still not satisfying. Only the inclusion of Leu led to the best FPF and FPD values (Aquino, Prota et al. 2012). Among all formulation, GISO3-Leu15 showed very satisfying aerodynamic properties as proven by FPF 49.4% and FPD of 50.4 mg (Table 2), values evaluated by Turbospin® device, a single-unit dose inhaler designed and patented by PH&T for effective drug delivery to the lungs.

Stability tests, performed storing the powders in a climatic chamber for 6 months at 25 ± 2 °C/60 ± 5% RH, were conducted to control over time hygroscopicity and dispersibility of G/Leu systems. After 6 month storage, no variation in powder weight was observed, GS content remained unaltered and no GS degradation product was recorded by HPLC analyses of aged powders.

In order to establish whether the particle engineering has any cytotoxic or cytostatic effect on bronchial epithelial cells (Zabner, Karp et al. 2003; Dechecchi, Nicolis et al. 2008), CuFi1 cells were treated for 24 h with increasing concentrations (from 0.0002 to 2 μM expressed as GS content) of GISO3 or GISO-Leu15 powders in comparison to raw GS. Results showed neither raw GS nor its formulations generally inhibited cells viability as determined by MTT assay (Figure 3b). Only raw GS at concentrations higher than 0.02 μM showed a slight but significant decrease in cell survival. An interesting observation is that an increase in Leu content up to 15%, as in GISO3-Leu15, faintly but not significantly decreased CuFi1 viability at concentration ranging from 0.02 to 0.2 μM (P<0.05) (Figure 3b) whereas at 2.0 μM did not. As previously observed in formulations for inhalation containing leucine (Prota, Santoro et al. 2011), this effect seems to be related to Leu ability to improve cell proliferation and metabolism of bronchial epithelial CF cells.

Furthermore ELISA BrdU immunoassay confirmed that raw GS slightly reduced CF cell growth only at the highest concentration (2 μM, P<0.01) (Figure 3a).

Therefore, G/Leu systems had no cytotoxic or cytostatic effect on CF epithelial lung cells (CuFi1 model), at concentrations up to 2 μM.

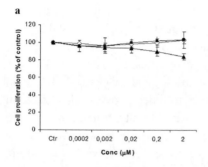
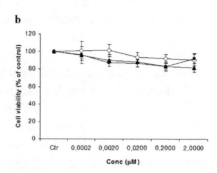

Figure 3. Effect of Gentamicin and its DPI formulations on CuFi1 cell proliferation and viability. Cells were treated for 24 h with: raw Gentamicin (raw GS, ▲), spray-dried Gentamicin (GISO3 ◊) and GS co-sprayed with 15%w/w leucine (GISO3-Leu15 ■) at concentrations from 0.0002 μM to 2 μM. Cell growth (a) was determined using a colorimetric bromodeoxyuridine (BrdU) cell proliferation ELISA kit. Cell viability (b) was determined by MTT assay. All data are shown as mean ± SD of three independent experiments, each done in duplicate (*P<0.05 and **P<0.01 vs control).

Finally, to verify the ability of the produced formulations to control *P. aeruginosa* infection, two different microbiological assays were performed. Preliminarily, microsystems were tested by a disc diffusion assay at a concentration corresponding to 5 μg of GS. Results showed that each powder produced an inhibition zone of growth with a diameter of about 2 cm, similar to that observed for GS raw material (Russo, Stigliani et al. 2013). Therefore, neither the spray drying process, nor the presence of the excipient seems to influence the antipseudomonal activity.

However, clinical identification of *P. aeruginosa* often includes identifying the secretion of pigments such as pyocianin (blue-green). In order to evaluate antibiotic activity of the formulations in a model which better reproduces pulmonary environment and, thus, may be clinically relevant, a modified pyocyanin assay was performed in presence of artificial mucus model (AM), developed taking into account CF mucus composition and characteristics (Russo, Stigliani et al. 2013). Results of our study confirmed that the growth of *P. aeruginosa* was inhibited equally by all formulations and in a manner comparable to neat gentamicin spray dried (G). Therefore, neither the spray drying process, nor the presence of the excipient seems to influence the antipseudomonal activity.

The formulation study of the "old" drug, gentamicin, demonstrate that the engineering process by spray drying, use of water-co-solvent systems as liquid feed and low rate of a safe excipient have enabled to obtain the required significant improvement in therapeutic GS performance. Identifying problems related to GS hygroscopicity and stickiness and reducing them by appropriate operations, led to obtain the specified performance goal, i.e. stable and aerosolizable microparticles in dry powder form for inhalation with an excellent emitted dose and good aerodynamic properties.

Particles engineering has not impact on biological properties of GS; in fact, GS/Leu engineered particles show no cytotoxic or cytostatic effect on bronchial epithelial cells bearing a CFTR F508/F508 mutant genotype and are able to preserve the antibiotic activity against *P. aeruginosa*, even in the presence of mucus. These findings together with the well known GS antibiotic activity and ability to partially restore CFTR expression in class I nonsense mutation, support the use of GS/Leu DPI as a valid alternative to common antibiotics already used in the management of Pa infections.

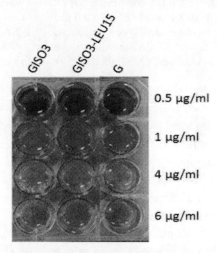

Figure 4. Modified pyocyanin assay on G dry powders. *P. aeruginosa* was cultured for 24h at 37°C in AM; powder concentration tested corresponded to 0.5, 1, 4 and 6 µg/ml of gentamicin used as control. The green color virulence factor pyocyanin decreases with the increase of GS concentrations.

2.2. Supercritical Fluid Technologies

A new approach in particle engineering developed to obtain micro/nanoparticles with desired characteristics is represented by the supercritical fluid (SCF) technology (Pasquali, Bettini et al. 2008; Tabernero, Martín del Valle et al. 2012). A SCF can be defined as any fluid which is at conditions above its critical point. Carbon dioxide, because of its accessible critical point at 31°C and 74 bar, and its low cost and non-toxicity, is the most widely used solvent in many SCF processes (Sihvonen, Järvenpää et al. 1999). Its critical temperature makes SCF suitable for processing heat-labile solutes at conditions close to room temperature.

A SCF can be used as: a solvent, in the rapid expansion of supercritical solutions (RESS); an antisolvent, in the supercritical antisolvent precipitation (SAS); a solute, in the particle from gas saturated solution (PGSS) (Reverchon and Antonacci 2007). Several papers and reviews have been published on pharmaceutical processing using these techniques (Carstensen 2001; Kompella and Koushik 2001; Kakumanu and Bansal 2003; Kayrak, Akman et al. 2003; York, Kompella et al. 2004). Recently, SC-CO_2-assisted spray drying techniques, such as CAN-BD (Carbon Dioxide Assisted Nebulization with a Bubble Dryer®) and SAA (Supercritical Assisted Atomization), have been proposed to produce micro- and nanoparticles of controlled size and distribution (Pasquali, Bettini et al. 2008). These techniques are aerosolization-based methods where supercritical CO_2 is used to assist the nebulization of the feed solution. The mechanism of the process is similar to micronization by spray drying: the SCF and the solution are intimately mixed and sprayed in a drying atmosphere. Claimed advantages of this process include the minimal decomposition of thermally labile drugs, the absence of a high-pressure vessel, and the small size of the produced particles (Charbit, Badens et al. 2004; Pasquali, Bettini et al. 2008).

2.2.1. Supercritical Assisted Atomization

SAA technology is a process based on the solubilization of controlled quantities of SC-CO_2 in liquid feeds containing a solid solute and on the subsequent atomization of the ternary solution through a nozzle. Therefore, SC-CO_2 plays both as co-solute being miscible with the solution to be treated, as well as pneumatic agent to atomize the solution in fine droplets (Reverchon 2002; Reverchon 2007). The solubilization is obtained in a packed bed saturator characterized by a high specific surface and large residence times. The solution formed in the saturator is, then, sent to a thin wall injector and sprayed into the precipitator at atmospheric pressure in a warm N_2 environment at fixed temperature. A two steps atomization is obtained: the primary droplets produced at the outlet of the injector (pneumatic atomization) are further divided in secondary droplets by CO_2 expansion from the inside of the primary ones (decompressive atomization). Then, the secondary droplets are rapidly dried by warm N_2 causing the micrometric and sub-micrometric particle precipitation. One of the most important aspects of SAA with respect to other SCF-based processes is that not only organic solvents, but also water and aqueous solutions can be used (Reverchon and Antonacci 2006).

Various studies have demonstrated that this technique can be successfully applied to the micronization of some pharmaceutical compounds obtaining particles in the range of 1-3 μm with controlled size distributions (Reverchon, Della Porta et al. 2004; Della Porta, Ercolino et al. 2006; Della Porta and Reverchon 2008). SAA has been also applied to the production of microparticulate drug delivery systems. Particularly, Reverchon et al., have successfully processed by SAA chitosan, hydroxypropyl methylcellulose, and cyclodextrins, obtaining, at the optimal process conditions, well-defined spherical microparticles with controlled drug release properties (Reverchon and Antonacci 2006; Reverchon and Antonacci 2007; Reverchon, Lamberti et al. 2008).

Therefore, selecting the right excipients and optimizing the operating conditions it is possible to tailor the SAA produced particles for different pharmaceutical applications.

2.2.2. Novel Gentamicin Topical Dosage Forms for Treatment of Wound Infections

Infections can be associated to many traumatic occurrences such as skin tears and burns or chronic pathologies or even to post-surgery complications (Baranoski and Ayello 2011). The main goal in treating the various types of wound infections should be to reduce the bacterial load in the wound to a level at which healing processes can take place (Baranoski 2008). Conventional systemic delivery of antibiotics, for both prevention and curing, suffers of the drawbacks of systemic toxicity with associated renal and liver complications, poor penetration into ischemic and necrotic tissue typical of post-traumatic and postoperative tissue and need for hospitalized monitoring (Campton-Johnston and Wilson 2001).

Alternative local delivery of antibiotics by topical administration, or even better by a local delivery device, may consent local control of infection while minimizing side effects and induced bacterial resistance (Persson, Salvi et al. 2006; Aviv, Berdicevsky et al. 2007; Boateng, Matthews et al. 2008).

A local antibiotic release profile should exhibit a high initial release rate in order to respond to the elevated risk of infection from bacteria introduced during the initial shock, followed by a sustained release at an effective level for inhibiting the occurrence of latent infection (Wu and Grainger 2006). Indeed, the effectiveness of wound controlled release devices is strongly dependent on the rate and manner in which the specific antibiotic is released. If it is released quickly, the entire amount could be released before the infection is arrested. If the release is delayed, infection may set in further, thus making it difficult to manage the wound. Finally, the release of antibiotics at levels below the Minimum Inhibitory Concentration (MIC) must be avoided because it may evoke bacterial resistance at the release site and intensify infectious complications (Gold and Moellering 1996; Aviv, Berdicevsky et al. 2007). Antibiotics of different families have been incorporated in controlled-release medical devices such as gentamicin, vancomycin, tobramycin, cefamandol, cephalothin, carbenicillin, amoxicillin etc. (Stigter, Bezemer et al. 2004; Zilberman and Elsner 2008) and various biodegradable devices have been produced using different processes (Blanco-Prieto, Lecaroz et al. 2002). In an preliminary research (Della Porta, Adami et al. 2010), SAA has been exploited not only as a micronization method but also as a thermal coagulation process for the production of gentamicin/albumin microspheres with slow drug release for the treatment of wound infections. More recently, we have proposed (Aquino, Auriemma et al. 2013), SAA technique for the development of specific controlled release microsystems, made by alginate, pectin and GS. Among natural polymers, two dextrans like alginate and pectin are known as wound dressing materials enhancing the healing process by maintaining optimal moist environment and via a direct effect on wound macrophages. Unlike other polymers, they can adhere to wound site (Fletcher 2005), absorb exudate by changing their physical state into a hydrogel able to cover and preserve an appropriate moisture at the wound bed (Baranoski 2008) while allowing effective oxygen circulation able to increase cells and tissues regeneration and lowering bacterial load (Boateng, Matthews et al. 2008). Moreover, alginate may induce cytokine production by human monocytes via an interaction with mannuronic residues of alginic acid. The pro-inflammatory stimulus is considered particularly useful in the treatment of chronic wounds, when macrophages have not achieved an appropriate differentiation state; the healing process could take advantage of exogenous pro-inflammatory stimuli to which macrophages are receptive (Thomas, Harding et al. 2000).

Therefore, the primary aim of our research was to design microencapsulate GS in such dextrans using SAA with the goal to be directly administered or charged in specific fibers or gels for wound dressing. As well known, the major concern when developing such drug delivery system is to control the technological and biopharmaceutical properties of the final product and to assure biological availability of the drug. Thus, the designed process comprises the study of the effects of i) the selected microencapsulation technique, ii) drug/polymers ratio, iii) operating conditions (i.e. feed composition and process parameters) on particle micromeritics (i.e., morphology, dimensional distribution, solid state of the loaded drug), drug release behavior, and GS antibiotic activity. In this chapter we report the best results obtained (Tables 3-4).

GS/alginate/pectin (GAP 1-4) particles, processed starting from aqueous solutions, were obtained as white powders made by microparticles with good spherical shape and uniform morphology (Figure 5). By contrast, as previously reported (Della Porta et al., 2010), when pure GS aqueous solutions were processed by SAA, pale yellow powder was obtained due to the partial degradation of GS in the precipitator. This observation suggests that the polymer blend consisting of alginate and pectin acts as a protecting agent, covering GS and avoiding its thermal degradation during microencapsulation process. Moreover, the increased stability of the SAA encapsulated GS, may also be due to its selective interaction, as a cationic drug, with mannuronic residues of the alginate (Iannuccelli, Coppi et al. 1996) by forming a polyelectrolyte complex. This hypothesis has been then confirmed by DSC (Differential Scanning Calorimetry) and FT-IR studies (Aquino, Auriemma et al. 2013).

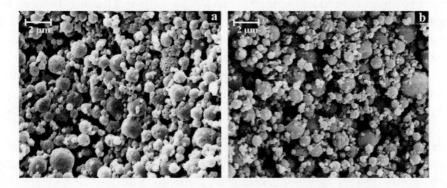

Figure 5. SEM images of GAP microparticles obtained by SAA at different GS/alginate/pectin ratio: GAP1 (a) and GAP4 (b).

Table 3. Composition and particle size distributions data of GAP microparticles produced by SAA at different GS/polymer blend ratio

Sample code	GS/Alginate/Pectin ratio (p/p/p)	Feed (w/v)	Mean diameter (μm)	d_{10} (μm)	d_{50} (μm)	d_{90} (μm)
GAP1	1:1:1	0.5%	2.12	0.89	1.91	3.51
GAP2	1:1:1	1.0%	2.15	0.91	1.82	3.62
GAP3	1:3:1	0.5%	1.71	0.70	1.45	3.09
GAP4	1:3:1	1.0%	1.75	0.73	1.39	3.14

As shown in table 3, GS/polymers ratio affected mean diameter and particle size distribution. Particularly, mean diameter increase from about 1.7 to 2.1 μm, according to the increase in GS/polymers ratio from 1:3:1 (GAP3-GAP4) to 1:1:1 (GAP1-GAP2).

Process yield, drug content, encapsulation efficiency and moisture content of GAP microspheres are reported in table 4. Process yield was satisfying ranging from 65 to 74% and encapsulation efficiency was over 100%. This phenomenon might be dependent on the previously described slight loss of polymers into the saturator, due to the so-called anti-solvent effect. In fact, the addition of carbon dioxide, before the microparticles formation into the precipitation chamber, can induce the precipitation of small quantities of polymer from the feed solution (Reverchon and De Marco 2006).

Table 4. Process yield and properties of GAP microparticles produced by SAA at different GS/polymer blend ratio. Each value represents the mean ± S.D. (n=3)

Sample code	Process yield (%)	Drug content (%)	E.E. (%)	Water content (%)	Drug content* (%)	Water content* (%)
GAP1	74±1.21	35.08±0.36	> 100	5.13±0.24	33.46±0.42	5.86±0.54
GAP2	68±1.09	39.38±0.60	> 100	4.65±0.25	37.89±0.54	5.01±0.42
GAP3	70±1.18	21.24±0.18	> 100	4.98±0.32	19.66±0.21	5.01±0.21
GAP4	65±1.08	29.63±0.09	> 100	4.43±0.21	28.94±0.17	4.56±0.28

*Values registered after 3 months in accelerated storage conditions; e.e. = encapsulation efficiency.

Stability tests, according to ICH accelerated storage conditions, were conducted to verify the stability of GS entrapped in the polymeric matrix by

SAA. As shown in table 4, even after harsh storage conditions, GS content was preserved and only a very slight increase in water uptake was detected for all GAP microparticles, whereas pure GS and SAA processed GS were deliquescent products.

As well known, powders' flow properties may influence the possibility to charge microparticles into fibers or wound dressing material or to spread the powder directly on a wound. Thus, the flowability of powders obtained by SAA was evaluated as ratio between bulk density (ρB) and tapped density (ρT): the lower is this ratio, the lower is flowability. Results indicated that $\rho B/\rho T$ ratio decreases from 0.50 (GAP2) to 0.45 (GAP3) and 0.41 (GAP 4), in accordance with their reduction in the mean diameter. Only GAP1 $\rho B/\rho T$ ratio (0.43) was found to be lower than expected; however, this phenomenon can be explained by considering the high surface roughness, partially collapsed and porous structure of GAP1 microparticles (Figure 5a), decreasing flowability of this formulation (Kawashima, Serigano et al. 1998).

The release behavior of the entrapped drug was monitored using vertical Franz-type diffusion cells. Figure 6 reports the permeation curves of both GAP microsystems and, as comparison, the permeation profile of pure GS processed by SAA. As expected for a BCS (Biopharmaceutical Classification System) class III drug, permeation of pure GS is a free diffusion process and total release of the drug is achieved in less than 3 hours. By contrast, GAP microparticles exhibit a prolonged release of the antibiotic following a non-fickian diffusion mechanism (Korsmeyer-Peppas equation with $0.62<n<0.69$) due to the swelling and erosion of the polymers that act as a barrier delaying drug release (Korsmeyer, Gurny et al. 1983).

The complete permeation of GS from GAP microparticles was achieved between 3 and 6 days, according to the increasing polymer blend concentration, while an initial burst effect (till 6 hours) was observed for all formulations. Such intensive release of GS in the first 6 hours of administration could be suitable to prevent infection spreading at the beginning of a local antibiotic therapy.

The antimicrobial activity of the developed formulations against *Staphylococcus aureus* was evaluated by both agar diffusion and time-killing assay (Aquino, Auriemma et al. 2013). Particularly, time-killing assay indicate that, the activity of GS is preserved at 6 days and higher at 12 and 24 days (Figure 7).

In view of these results, it is possible to conclude that the formulation study of the "old" drug, gentamicin, demonstrate that the engineering process by Supercritical Assisted Atomization and use of dextran carriers may successfully produce dextran based microsystems with high gentamicin content and encapsulation efficiency. Identifying problems related to GS hygroscopicity and instability, and reducing them by appropriate operations led to the improvement in technological properties of the final powder and to a drug prolonged release.

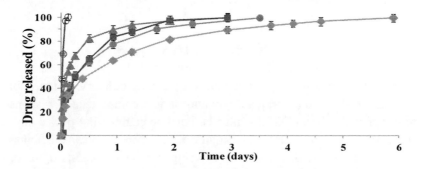

Figure 6. Release profiles of GAP microparticles manufactured by SAA: GAP1 (-●-), GAP2 (-▲-), GAP3 (-■-) and GAP4 (-◆-) in comparison with pure GS produced by SAA (-○-). Mean ± SD; (n=6).

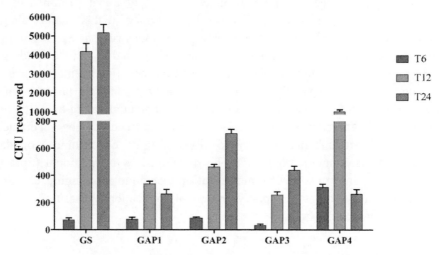

Figure 7. Antimicrobial activity of GAP1-4 against *Staphylococcus aureus* after 6, 12 and 24 days of incubation by time-killing test. GAP1-4 are used at concentrations corresponding to 1.5 mg/ml of gentamicin used as control; CFU recovered = number of *S. aureus colony forming unit*.

Particles engineering also by SAA has not impact on biological properties of GS which activity is retained. The initial burst effect followed by a GS prolonged release suggests that GAP microsystems may be proposed as interesting candidates to be loaded in wound dressing preparations such as fibers and gels or to be administered as self-consistent formulations overstaying wounds.

CONCLUSION

Today, there is a strong need for innovative drug delivery systems able to maximize "new" or "old" drug activity and patient compliance in response to current therapeutic and clinical demands. Particle engineering play a key role in the development of effective, safe and patient-friendly new medicines. In fact, as above discussed, particle engineering approach consists of precisely identify problems of a drug and health need, create and develop a solution that solves the problems or meets the need, defines particle attributes such as narrow particle-size distribution, improved dispersibility, enhanced drug stability, with the goal to optimize bioavailability, obtain a sustained drug release and/or precise targeting. The results presented in this chapter show how particle engineering via two interesting techniques such as Spray Drying and Supercritical Assisted Atomization can be applied to an "old" drug, gentamicin sulfate, to develop new drug delivery systems which meets current therapeutic input and health demands. Accurately planning a product with specified performance goal may led to exploit the potential and re-evaluate the use of an old-generation antibiotic addressing current need of new medicines effective against infections in cystic fibrosis (CF) or chronic wounds. Gentamicin-based microparticles may be developed by a traditional (Spray-drying) or an innovative (SAA) micronization technique and administered by alternative route such as pulmonary or topical application bypassing its well known oto- and nephro-toxicity.

REFERENCES

Abdelghany, S. M., D. J. Quinn, et al. (2012). "Gentamicin-loaded nanoparticles show improved antimicrobial effects towards Pseudomonas aeruginosa infection." *Int J Nanomedicine* 7: 4053-4063.

Aquino, R. P., G. Auriemma, et al. (2013). "Design and production of gentamicin/dextrans microparticles by supercritical assisted atomisation for the treatment of wound bacterial infections." *Int J Pharm* 440(2): 188-194.

Aquino, R. P., L. Prota, et al. (2012). "Dry powder inhalers of gentamicin and leucine: formulation parameters, aerosol performance and in vitro toxicity on CuFi1 cells." *Int J Pharm* 426(1-2): 100-107.

Aviv, M., I. Berdicevsky, et al. (2007). "Gentamicin-loaded bioresorbable films for prevention of bacterial infections associated with orthopedic implants." *J Biomed Mater Res A* 83(1): 10-19.

Balakumar, P., A. Rohilla, et al. (2010). "Gentamicin-induced nephrotoxicity: Do we have a promising therapeutic approach to blunt it?" *Pharmacological Research* 62(3): 179-186.

Balmayor, E. R., E. T. Baran, et al. (2012). "Injectable biodegradable starch/chitosan delivery system for the sustained release of gentamicin to treat bone infections." *Carbohydr Polym* 87(1): 8-8.

Baranoski, S. (2008). "Choosing a wound dressing, part 1." *Nursing* 38(1): 60-61.

Baranoski, S. (2008). "Choosing a wound dressing, part 2." *Nursing* 38(2): 14-15.

Baranoski, S. and E. Ayello (2011). *Wound Care Essentials: Practice Principles*, Wolter Kluwer Health, Lippincott Williams & Wilkins.

Blanco-Prieto, M., C. Lecaroz, et al. (2002). "In vitro evaluation of gentamicin released from microparticles." *Int J Pharm* 242(1-2): 203-206.

Boateng, J. S., K. H. Matthews, et al. (2008). "Wound healing dressings and drug delivery systems: A review." *Journal of Pharmaceutical Sciences* 97(8): 2892-2923.

Boraey, M. A., S. Hoe, et al. (2013). "Improvement of the dispersibility of spray-dried budesonide powders using leucine in an ethanol–water cosolvent system." *Powder Technology* 236(0): 171-178.

Buttini, F., P. Colombo, et al. (2012). "Particles and powders: tools of innovation for non-invasive drug administration." *J Control Release* 161(2): 693-702.

Campton-Johnston, S. and J. Wilson (2001). "Infected wound management: advanced technologies, moisture-retentive dressings, and die-hard methods." *Crit Care Nurs* Q 24(2): 64-77.

Carstensen, J. T. (2001). *Advanced pharmaceutical solids*, CRC Press.

Charbit, G., E. Badens, et al. (2004). Supercritical Fluid Technology for Drug Product Development, Drugs and Pharmaceutical Sciences, vol. 138, Marcel Dekker Inc., New York.

Chew, N. Y. and H. K. Chan (2002). "The role of particle properties in pharmaceutical powder inhalation formulations." *J Aerosol Med* 15(3): 325-330.

Chew, N. Y., B. Y. Shekunov, et al. (2005). "Effect of amino acids on the dispersion of disodium cromoglycate powders." *J Pharm Sci* 94(10): 2289-2300.

Chow, A. H., H. H. Tong, et al. (2007). "Particle engineering for pulmonary drug delivery." *Pharm Res* 24(3): 411-437.

Clancy, J. P., Z. Bebok, et al. (2001). "Evidence that systemic gentamicin suppresses premature stop mutations in patients with cystic fibrosis." *Am J Respir Crit Care Med* 163(7): 1683-1692.

Coelho, J. F., P. C. Ferreira, et al. (2010). "Drug delivery systems: Advanced technologies potentially applicable in personalized treatments." *Epma* J 1(1): 164-209.

Davis, B. D. (1987). "Mechanism of bactericidal action of aminoglycosides." *Microbiol Rev* 51(3): 341-350.

de Jesús Valle, M. J., F. G. López, et al. (2007). "Pulmonary versus Systemic Delivery of Antibiotics: Comparison of Vancomycin Dispositions in the Isolated Rat Lung." *Antimicrobial Agents and Chemotherapy* 51(10): 3771-3774.

Dechecchi, M. C., E. Nicolis, et al. (2008). "Anti-inflammatory effect of miglustat in bronchial epithelial cells." *J Cyst Fibros* 7(6): 555-565.

Della Porta, G., R. Adami, et al. (2010). "Albumin/gentamicin microspheres produced by supercritical assisted atomization: optimization of size, drug loading and release." *J Pharm Sci* 99(11): 4720-4729.

Della Porta, G., S. F. Ercolino, et al. (2006). "Corticosteroid microparticles produced by supercritical-assisted atomization: process optimization, product characterization, and "in vitro" performance." *J Pharm Sci* 95(9): 2062-2076.

Della Porta, G. and E. Reverchon (2008). "Supercritical Fluid-Based Technologies for Particulate Drug Delivery." *Handbook of Particulate Drug Delivery* 1.

Depreter, F., G. Pilcer, et al. (2013). "Inhaled proteins: challenges and perspectives." *Int J Pharm* 447(1-2): 251-280.

Du, M., J. R. Jones, et al. (2002). "Aminoglycoside suppression of a premature stop mutation in a Cftr-/- mouse carrying a human CFTR-G542X transgene." *J Mol Med (Berl)* 80(9): 595-604.

Fletcher, J. (2005). "Understanding wound dressings: alginates." *Nurs Times* 101(16): 53-54.

Forge, A. and J. Schacht (2000). "Aminoglycoside antibiotics." *Audiol Neurootol* 5(1): 3-22.

Friebel, C., H. Steckel, et al. (2012). "Rational design of a dry powder inhaler: device design and optimisation." *J Pharm Pharmacol* 64(9): 1303-1315.

Gold, H. S. and R. C. Moellering, Jr. (1996). "Antimicrobial-drug resistance." *N Engl J Med* 335(19): 1445-1453.

Gonzalez, L. S., 3rd and J. P. Spencer (1998). "Aminoglycosides: a practical review." *Am Fam Physician* 58(8): 1811-1820.

Haswani, D. K., H. Nettey, et al. (2006). "Formulation, characterization and pharmacokinetic evaluation of gentamicin sulphate loaded albumin microspheres." *J Microencapsul* 23(8): 875-886.

Hu, T., H. Zhao, et al. (2008). "Engineering Pharmaceutical Fine Particles of Budesonide for Dry Powder Inhalation (DPI)." *Ind. Eng. Chem. Res.* 47(23): 9623-9627.

Iannuccelli, V., G. Coppi, et al. (1996). "Biodegradable intraoperative system for bone infection treatment II. In vivo evaluation." *International Journal of Pharmaceutics* 143(2): 187-194.

Islam, N. and M. J. Cleary (2012). "Developing an efficient and reliable dry powder inhaler for pulmonary drug delivery – A review for multidisciplinary researchers." *Medical Engineering & Physics* 34(4): 409-427.

Islam, N. and E. Gladki (2008). "Dry powder inhalers (DPIs)--a review of device reliability and innovation." *Int J Pharm* 360(1-2): 1-11.

Ito, Y., T. Kusawake, et al. (2005). "Oral solid gentamicin preparation using emulsifier and adsorbent." *J Control Release* 105(1-2): 23-31.

Joshi, J. T. (2011). " Review on Micronization Techniques." Journal of *Pharmaceutical Science and Technology* 3(7): 651-681.

Kakumanu, V. K. and A. K. Bansal (2003). "Supercritical fluid technology in pharmaceutical research." *Crips* 4(1): 8-12.

Kawashima, Y., T. Serigano, et al. (1998). "Effect of surface morphology of carrier lactose on dry powder inhalation property of pranlukast hydrate." *International Journal of Pharmaceutics* 172(1–2): 179-188.

Kayrak, D., U. Akman, et al. (2003). "Micronization of Ibuprofen by RESS." *The Journal of Supercritical Fluids* 26(1): 17-31.

Kompella, U. B. and K. Koushik (2001). "Preparation of drug delivery systems using supercritical fluid technology." *Crit Rev Ther Drug Carrier Syst* 18(2): 173-199.

Korsmeyer, R. W., R. Gurny, et al. (1983). "Mechanisms of solute release from porous hydrophilic polymers." *International Journal of Pharmaceutics* 15(1): 25-35.

Krasko, M. Y., J. Golenser, et al. (2007). "Gentamicin extended release from an injectable polymeric implant." *Journal of Controlled Release* 117(1): 90-96.

Labiris, N. R. and M. B. Dolovich (2003). "Pulmonary drug delivery. Part I: Physiological factors affecting therapeutic effectiveness of aerosolized medications." *British Journal of Clinical Pharmacology* 56(6): 588-599.

Lechuga-Ballesteros, D., C. Charan, et al. (2008). "Trileucine improves aerosol performance and stability of spray-dried powders for inhalation." *J Pharm Sci* 97(1): 287-302.

Li, H. Y., P. C. Seville, et al. (2005). "The use of amino acids to enhance the aerosolisation of spray-dried powders for pulmonary gene therapy." *J Gene Med* 7(3): 343-353.

Maas, S. G., G. Schaldach, et al. (2011). "The impact of spray drying outlet temperature on the particle morphology of mannitol." *Powder Technology* 213(1–3): 27-35.

Mack, P., K. Horvath, et al. (2012). "Particle engineering for inhalation formulation and delivery of therapeutics." *Liquidia Inhalation Magazin.*

Mendelman, P. M., A. L. Smith, et al. (1985). "Aminoglycoside penetration, inactivation, and efficacy in cystic fibrosis sputum." *Am Rev Respir Dis* 132(4): 761-765.

Mugabe, C., A. O. Azghani, et al. (2005). "Liposome-mediated gentamicin delivery: development and activity against resistant strains of Pseudomonas aeruginosa isolated from cystic fibrosis patients." *J Antimicrob Chemother* 55(2): 269-271.

Mukhopadhyay, S., M. Singh, et al. (1996). "Nebulised antipseudomonal antibiotic therapy in cystic fibrosis: a meta-analysis of benefits and risks." *Thorax* 51(4): 364-368.

Padhi, B. K., M. B. Chougule, et al. (2006). "Optimization of formulation components and characterization of large respirable powders containing high therapeutic payload." *Pharm Dev Technol* 11(4): 465-475.

Paolino, D., P. Sinha, et al. (2006). Drug Delivery Systems. Encyclopedia of *Medical Devices and Instrumentation*, John Wiley & Sons, Inc.

Parikh, D. M. (2011). "Recent Advances in Particle Engineering for Pharmaceutical Applications." *American Pharmaceutical Review* Volume 14(2).

Parlati, C., P. Colombo, et al. (2009). "Pulmonary spray dried powders of tobramycin containing sodium stearate to improve aerosolization efficiency." *Pharm Res* 26(5): 1084-1092.

Pasquali, I., R. Bettini, et al. (2008). "Supercritical fluid technologies: An innovative approach for manipulating the solid-state of pharmaceuticals." *Advanced Drug Delivery Reviews* 60(3): 399-410.

Persson, G. R., G. E. Salvi, et al. (2006). "Antimicrobial therapy using a local drug delivery system (Arestin®) in the treatment of peri-implantitis. I: microbiological outcomes." *Clinical Oral Implants Research* 17(4): 386-393.

Pilcer, G. and K. Amighi (2010). "Formulation strategy and use of excipients in pulmonary drug delivery." *Int J Pharm* 392(1-2): 1-19.

Prayle, A. and A. R. Smyth (2010). "Aminoglycoside use in cystic fibrosis: therapeutic strategies and toxicity." *Curr Opin Pulm Med* 16(6): 604-610.

Prota, L., A. Santoro, et al. (2011). "Leucine enhances aerosol performance of naringin dry powder and its activity on cystic fibrosis airway epithelial cells." *Int J Pharm* 412(1-2): 8-19.

Rabbani, N. R. and P. C. Seville (2005). "The influence of formulation components on the aerosolisation properties of spray-dried powders." *J Control Release* 110(1): 130-140.

Ramsey, B. W., M. S. Pepe, et al. (1999). "Intermittent administration of inhaled tobramycin in patients with cystic fibrosis. Cystic Fibrosis Inhaled Tobramycin Study Group." *N Engl J Med* 340(1): 23-30.

Reverchon, E. (2002). "Supercritical-assisted atomization to produce micro- and/or nanoparticles of controlled size and distribution." *Industrial & engineering chemistry research* 41(10): 2405-2411.

Reverchon, E. (2007). Process for the production of micro and/or nano particles, Google Patents.

Reverchon, E. and A. Antonacci (2006). "Cyclodextrins micrometric powders obtained by supercritical fluid processing." *Biotechnol Bioeng* 94(4): 753-761.

Reverchon, E. and A. Antonacci (2007). "Polymer microparticles production by supercritical assisted atomization." *The Journal of Supercritical Fluids* 39(3): 444-452.

Reverchon, E. and I. De Marco (2006). "Supercritical fluid extraction and fractionation of natural matter." *The Journal of Supercritical Fluids* 38(2): 146-166.

Reverchon, E., G. Della Porta, et al. (2004). "Griseofulvin micronization and dissolution rate improvement by supercritical assisted atomization." *J Pharm Pharmacol* 56(11): 1379-1387.

Reverchon, E., G. Lamberti, et al. (2008). "Supercritical fluid assisted production of HPMC composite microparticles." *The Journal of Supercritical Fluids* 46(2): 185-196.

Russo, P., M. Stigliani, et al. (2013). "Gentamicin and leucine inhalable powder: what about antipseudomonal activity and permeation through cystic fibrosis mucus?" *Int J Pharm* 440(2): 250-255.

Selimoglu, E. (2007). "Aminoglycoside-induced ototoxicity." *Curr Pharm Des* 13(1): 119-126.

Seville, P. C., T. P. Learoyd, et al. (2007). "Amino acid-modified spray-dried powders with enhanced aerosolisation properties for pulmonary drug delivery." *Powder Technology* 178(1): 40-50.

Shoyele, S. A., N. Sivadas, et al. (2011). "The effects of excipients and particle engineering on the biophysical stability and aerosol performance of parathyroid hormone (1-34) prepared as a dry powder for inhalation." *AAPS PharmSciTech* 12(1): 304-311.

Shur, J., T. G. Nevell, et al. (2008). "Cospray-dried unfractionated heparin with L-leucine as a dry powder inhaler mucolytic for cystic fibrosis therapy." *J Pharm Sci* 97(11): 4857-4868.

Sihvonen, M., E. Järvenpää, et al. (1999). "Advances in supercritical carbon dioxide technologies." *Trends in Food Science & Technology* 10(6–7): 217-222.

Son, Y. J. and J. T. McConville (2008). "Advancements in dry powder delivery to the lung." *Drug Dev Ind Pharm* 34(9): 948-959.

Sou, T., E. N. Meeusen, et al. (2011). "New developments in dry powder pulmonary vaccine delivery." *Trends Biotechnol* 29(4): 191-198.

Stigter, M., J. Bezemer, et al. (2004). "Incorporation of different antibiotics into carbonated hydroxyapatite coatings on titanium implants, release and antibiotic efficacy." *J Control Release* 99(1): 127-137.

Tabernero, A., E. M. Martín del Valle, et al. (2012). "Supercritical fluids for pharmaceutical particle engineering: Methods, basic fundamentals and modelling." *Chemical Engineering and Processing: Process Intensification* 60(0): 9-25.

Telko, M. J. and A. J. Hickey (2005). "Dry powder inhaler formulation." *Respir Care* 50(9): 1209-1227.

Thomas, A., K. G. Harding, et al. (2000). "Alginates from wound dressings activate human macrophages to secrete tumour necrosis factor-alpha." *Biomaterials* 21(17): 1797-1802.

Tiwari, G., T. R., et al. (2012). "Drug delivery systems: An updated review." *Int J Pharm Investig.* 2(1): 2–11.

Vehring, R. (2008). "Pharmaceutical particle engineering via spray drying." *Pharm Res* 25(5): 999-1022.

Wilschanski, M., C. Famini, et al. (2000). "A pilot study of the effect of gentamicin on nasal potential difference measurements in cystic fibrosis patients carrying stop mutations." *Am J Respir Crit Care Med* 161(3 Pt 1): 860-865.

Wilschanski, M., Y. Yahav, et al. (2003). "Gentamicin-induced correction of CFTR function in patients with cystic fibrosis and CFTR stop mutations." *N Engl J Med* 349(15): 1433-1441.

Wu, P. and D. W. Grainger (2006). "Drug/device combinations for local drug therapies and infection prophylaxis." *Biomaterials* 27(11): 2450-2467.

Wu, X., D. J. Hayes, et al. (2013). "Design and physicochemical characterization of advanced spray-dried tacrolimus multifunctional particles for inhalation." *Drug Des Devel Ther* 7: 59-72.

York, P. Y., U. B. Kompella, et al. (2004). *Supecritical Fluid Technology for Drug Product Development,* CRC Press.

Zabner, J., P. Karp, et al. (2003). "Development of cystic fibrosis and noncystic fibrosis airway cell lines." *Am J Physiol Lung Cell Mol Physiol* 284(5): L844-854.

Zilberman, M. and J. J. Elsner (2008). "Antibiotic-eluting medical devices for various applications." *J Control Release* 130(3): 202-215.

In: Gentamicin
Editor: Emilie Kruger

ISBN: 978-1-62808-841-0
© 2013 Nova Science Publishers, Inc.

Chapter 3

USE OF NATURAL PRODUCTS TO ENHANCE THE ANTIBIOTIC ACTIVITY OF GENTAMICIN AND OTHER AMINOGLYCOSIDES: THE FUTURE OF ANTIBIOTIC THERAPY

Cícera Natalia Figueirêdo Leite Gondim[1],
Nadghia Figueiredo Leite[1], Jacqueline Cosmo Andrade[1],
Maria Flaviana Bezerra Morais-Braga[1],
Glaucia Morgana de Melo Guedes[1],
Saulo Relison Tintino[1], Cícera Cislânia Araújo Tavares[1],
Maria Audilene de Freitas[1],
Liscássia Beatriz Batista Alencar[1],
Celestina Elba Sobral de Souza[1],
Rosimeire Sabino Albuquerque[1],
Edinardo Fagner Ferreira Matias[1],
Francisco Assis Bezerra da Cunha[1],
Dara Isabel Vieira de Brito[1],
Anne Karyzia Lima Santos de Lavor[1],
João Victor de Alencar Ferreira[1],
Fernando Gomes Figueredo[1], Luciene Ferreira de Lima[1]
and Henrique Douglas Melo Coutinho[2]
[1]Departamento de Ciências Biológicas, [2]Departamento de Química
Biológica, Universidade Regional do Cariri, Crato, CE, Brasil

ABSTRACT

The capacity to develop resistance to antibacterial agents is a characteristic observed among microorganisms in general. Bacteria are able to develop different mechanisms of resistance, which are genetically coded, where resistance genes can be acquired through mutation and transfer of genetic material.

Essential oils consist of volatile elements, which are present in many plant organs, are related to various functions necessary for the survival of the plant, exerting a fundamental role in the defense against microorganisms and offering protection.

The use of extracts and essential oils of plants as antimicrobial agents shows a low possibility that microorganisms will acquire resistance to their action, because they are complex mixtures, making microbial adaptation very difficult.

The chapter discuss the activity of isolated substances isolated citronellol, citronellal and myrcene on bacterial resistance in combination with antibiotics using direct and gaseous contact methods.

Keywords: Resistant bacteria, Citronellol, Citronellal, Myrcene, Contant gaseous, Contact direct, Modulation

INTRODUCTION

Worldwide, there is a large number of bacterial strains resistant to multiple drugs, mainly in the hospital environment, increasing morbidity, inherent costs of health care, and rates of mortality due to infections as well [1]. In the field of medicine, indications for the use of antibacterials are divided into: prophylactic, therapeutic without knowledge of the infectious agent (empirical), and therapeutic with knowledge of the infectious agent and its sensitivity to antibiotics (guided use). In these situations, inadequacy can occur with respect to the use of the antibacterials, with unnecessary utilization or error in the choice of the type, dose, administration route and duration of the treatment [2]. Therefore, resistance is a phenomenon characterized not only by evolutionary pressure, but especially by the indiscriminate and irrational use of antibiotics in treatment [1].

Bacterial resistance can be transferred by various mechanisms, where it can occur between microorganisms of the same or different populations, such as from animal to human microbiota and vice versa. The development of bacterial resistance, besides determining lower drug efficacy, also represents a potential risk to public health [3].

The capacity to develop resistance to antibacterial agents is a characteristic observed among microorganisms in general. Meanwhile, bacteria are able to develop different mechanisms of resistance, which are genetically coded, where resistance genes can be acquired through mutation and transfer of genetic material [2].

The development of infections in humans includes a diversity of Gram-positive and -negative bacteria, as described below.

Bacteria of the genus *Staphylococcus* are distributed in nature, as well as in the normal microbiota of the skin and mucosa of animals and birds. Some species of *Staphylococcus* are often recognized as etiological agents of opportunistic infections in many animals and humans [4, 5]. *Staphylococcus aureus, S. epidermidis, S. saprophyticus* and *S. haemolyticus* are the species that are the most important causative agents of human infections. Besides causing different types of intoxications, *S. aureus* represents the most common etiological agent in infections such as furuncles, carbuncles, abscesses, myocarditis, endocarditis, pneumonia, meningitis and bacterial arthritis [6].

The species *Pseudomonas aeruginosa* is responsible for a variety of infections, such as those that attack the skin, urinary tract, ears and eyes. The wide environmental distribution of *Pseudomonas* is assured by its non-fastidious requirements for growth, besides having numerous structural factors, enzymes and toxins that potentiate its virulence, as well as making it resistant to the more common antibiotics [7].

Escherichia coli is one of the principal causes of infectious diseases in humans. It is known for its production of enterotoxins, whose properties and participation in diarrhea have been widely investigated. The activity of its cytotoxins and their role in human infection have been identified [8, 9], mainly in infections of the urinary tract [10].

A progression of the antibiotic resistance of *Klebsiella pneumoniae* is a great concern, with the appearance of *K. pneumonia,* a producer of extended spectrum beta-lactamase (ESBL), a class of enzymes that confer resistance to all the cephalosporins [11], causing outbreaks in neonatal intensive care units [12]. *K. pneumoniae* is known by many clinicians as the cause of community-acquired pneumonia, occurring mainly in immunocompromised patients.

With regard to the growing importance given to bacterial infections in hospital communities and the progressive development of the antimicrobial resistance, a large number of studies have been conducted with natural products seeking a new perspective in the treatment of bacterial infections.

The first descriptions of medicinal plants by humans appeared in sacred scriptures in the Ebers papyrus. They list about 100 diseases and describe a large number of drugs of animal and plant nature [13].

All the magical-sorcery empirism of the art of healing throughout the history of humanity, from snake oils to mandrakes, is found in Paracelsus (1493-1541), its most polemic figure. He proposed the theory the "Doctrine of Signatures," which states that the "pharmacological activity" of a plant is related to its morphological appearance. Thus, for example, the "serpentaria," herb of the family Araceae, whose twisted stem brings to mind the body of a snake, would serve as a cure for snakebites [13, 14].

The great navigations brought about the discovery of new continents, bequeathing the modern world a large therapeutic arsenal of plant origin up to now indispensable to medicine.

Medicinal plants are a recurrent theme on the agenda of Brazilian science. Brazilian chemists and pharmacologists with international reputations all agree that studies on medicinal plants in Brazil still do not receive the attention that they deserve from funding agencies. However, now there is a critical mass of qualified scientists in the areas of chemistry and pharmacology [15].

After the discovery of medications of plant origin, it is understandable that some transnational companies were interested in the search of new bioactive substances from natural products. This search was intensified in the 1990s, especially in the tropical forests, where a large part of biodiversity is concentrated, especially in Brazil, and where the great majority of their species still lack any chemical or biological study [13].

In the last decades, an important change in the paradigm of Western societies has led to plant products again assuming a leading role in health care for large contingents of populations in developing and developed countries.

1. MECHANISMS OF BACTERIAL RESISTANCE

The two main factors involved in the development of resistance to antibiotics in bacteria are selective pressure and the presence of resistance genes [16]. The genes that code for resistance to antimicrobials are localized in the chromosome or plasmids. Chromosomal DNA is relatively more stable, while plasmid DNA is easily transported from one strain to another by bacterial conjugation, allowing the transfer of genes including those of resistance to antimicrobials [17].

There are basically three mechanisms of bacterial resistance to antibacterials: enzymatic inactivation of the antibiotic; molecular modifications to prevent binding of the antibiotic to its binding site; and permeability barrier or modifications to prevent the antibiotic from reaching its target. It should be pointed out that these mechanisms can occur simultaneously [18].

The inactivation of the antibiotics by enzymes occurs among aminoglycosides [18]. The principal mechanism of resistance to aminoglycosides in staphylococci is the inactivation of the drugs by cellular enzymes that modify aminoglycosides. Various distinct *loci* that code for such drug-modifying enzymes were characterized in staphylococci. Clinically, the most important of these code for the enzymes acetyltransferase (AAC), adenylyltransferase (ANT) and phosphotransferase (APH). The amino-glycosides, with modifications to amino groups by AAC or to hydroxyl groups by ANT or APH, lose the ability to bind to ribosomes and then no longer inhibit protein synthesis in bacterial cells [19].

Enzymatic inactivation also occurs by means of enzymes called beta-lactamases. Beta-lactamases constitute a heterogeneous group of enzymes capable of inactivating penicillins, cephalosporins and sometimes monobactam. These enzymes are often produced by Gram-positive and Gram-negative bacteria, aerobic and anaerobic, and break the beta-lactam ring by irreversible hydroxylation of the amide bond, resulting in inactivation of the antibiotic. Although the final result of its action is the same, enzymatic activity is variable depending on the type of beta-lactamase produced and diverse existing substrates. There is variation in substrate specificity between beta-lactamases: some hydroxylate preferentially penicillins, others have an affinity for cephalosporins, and some enzymes inactivate both classes of antibiotics. Some pathogens produce different types of beta-lactamases, where different strains can produce different enzymes, or a single strain can produce more than one type of enzyme [20].

The molecular modifications to prevent the binding of the antibiotic to its binding site also occurs in beta-lactam antibiotics [21]. In this type of resistance, the bacterial cell develops a new penicillin-binding protein (PBP) through the substitution of an amino acid giving rise to PBP 2a, which differs from PBP, because it has a low affinity for beta-lactam antibiotics, where it is unable to bind the antibiotics effectively and to inhibit the synthesis of the cell wall [22].

This same type of resistance also occurs in quinolones, where the bacterial cell modifies the binding site of the antibiotic in DNA-DNA gyrase or topoisomerase II. The enzyme DNA-gyrase or topoisomerase II is a tetramer, consisting of two subunits coded by the gene gyrA and two b subunits coded by the gene gyrB. This enzyme is responsible for the supercoiling of bacterial DNA. The DNA-DNA gyrase complex is formed by covalent binding between the two, and a single turn is wrapped around the enzyme with the entrance and exit points located very close together [23, 24]. The inhibition of gyrase-DNA occurs by the cooperative binding between quinolones and DNA. When the enzyme breaks both DNA strands at the level of four base pairs, the drug inserts in the space between the non-paired bases. This binding impedes the later movement of the strands and fixes the enzyme, hindering it from continuing to exert its catalytic action. In the altered bacterial cell, this does not occur, because there is a modification of the binding site in the bacterial DNA gyrase [24].

Resistance to macrolides also results mainly from the modification of the binding site on the ribosome, i.e., more precisely on the 23S subunit of the ribosomal RNA [25, 26].

Modifications of the binding site also occur in sulfonamides. Sulfonamides are antibiotics that act by inhibiting dihydropteroato synthase, the enzyme responsible for linking p-aminobenzoic acid and pteridine in bacterial folic acid synthesis. Some Gram-negative bacilli synthesize via plasmid or transposon, an altered dihydropteroate synthase, that lacks affinity for sulfa drugs but maintains its biochemical activity in the production of folate. Without the inhibitory effect of sulfa drugs, bacteria grow normally, becoming resistant to the drugs. A similar mechanism affects trimethoprim, in the phase following the synthesis of folic acid, in its reduction to tetrahydrofolate by dihydrofolate reductase [27].

A permeability barrier or modifications to prevent the antibiotic from reaching its target is another type of mechanism of bacterial resistance. This is often associated with diminution of the permeability of the outer membrane of Gram-negative bacteria. The passage of molecules from inside the cell occurs depending on particular characteristics such as charge, structure and dimension and through membrane proteins (porins), which form channels. Antibiotics utilize this way to reach the interior of the bacterial cell or the periplasmic space as is the case of the β-lactam antibiotics. Thus, a loss of function of these proteins can effectively cause a decrease in susceptibility to a various antibiotics [28].

This type of route in the development of drug resistance includes as well efflux systems also known as efflux pumps [29]. The specificity of the antibiotic can vary depending on the efflux pump. Characterized by the active pumping of antimicrobials from the intracellular to extracellular environment, this mechanism produces bacterial resistance to particular antimicrobials, as is the case of the resistance to tetracyclines coded by plasmids in *E. coli,* due to the presence of integral proteins of the bacterial plasma membrane [30].

2. ANTIBACTERIAL ACTIVITY OF NATURAL PRODUCTS

With respect to the growing clinical importance given to the hospital community and bacterial infections and the progressive development of antimicrobial resistance, a great number of scientific studies have been conducted, focusing on the antibacterial properties of plant products [31, 32, 33]. Various plants have been evaluated not only to demonstrate their direct antimicrobial potential, but also as sources of substances with the potential of being agents capable of modifying antibiotic action [34, 35].

The use of extracts and essential oils of plants as antimicrobial agents shows a low possibility that microorganisms will acquire resistance to their action, because they are complex mixtures, making microbial adaptation very difficult [36].

The mechanisms by which extracts can inhibit the growth of microorganisms are varied, and can be due in part to the hydrophobic nature of some components. These components can interact with the lipid bilayer of the cell membrane and affect the respiratory chain and energy production [37] or even make the cell more permeable to antibiotics, leading to the interruption of vital cellular activity [38].

Interference with enzyme systems of bacteria can also be a potential mechanism of action [39]. These mechanisms of action can be achieved by the combination of antibiotics with extracts at sub-inhibitory concentrations applied directly to the culture medium [40, 41, 42].

This strategy is called "shotgun herbs" or "synergistic effect of various segments" and refers to the utilization of plants and drugs in an attempt to use mono- or multi-extract combinations, which can affect not only a single target, but various targets, where the different therapeutic components work together in a synergistic or antagonistic way. This approach is not only for combinations of extracts; combinations of natural products or extracts and synthetic products or antibiotics are also possible [43, 44].

Various works focusing on antibacterial activity and modulatory activity against antimicrobial resistance have been reported involving the species *Costus arabicus, Ocimum gratissimum, Eugenia jambolana, Eugeia uniflora* and *Hyptis* martiusi of the flora of the Araripe plateau located in Crato - Ceara-Brazil [5, 45, 46].

3. ESSENTIAL OILS

Essential oils consist of volatile elements, which are present in many plant organs, are related to various functions necessary for the survival of the plant, exerting a fundamental role in the defense against microorganisms and offering protection [47, 46] in the actions of allopathic treatments [49]. They have been known and utilized since ancient times because of their biological properties, especially antibacterial, antifungal and antioxidant [50].

The majority of the biological activities exhibited by medicinal plants are attributed to products of secondary metabolism [51]. Essential oils show a wide spectrum of inhibitory activity already proven against fungi and bacteria [52]. The isolation of the first pure substances of the plant kingdom began in the XVIII century. This century, along with the XIX, is characterized by works in extraction, mainly of organic acids and alkaloids. It was in this era that morphine (1806), quinine and strychnine (1820) were isolated [13].

Citronellol

Citronellol (Fig. 1) is an excellent air freshner and insect repellent, besides having a local antimicrobial and acaricidal action [53]. Citronellol is extracted from various plants, such as lemongrass (*Cymbopogon nardus*) [54], tangerine (*Citrus reticulata*), citronella grass (*Cymbopogon winterianus*), palmarosa (*Cymbopogon martinii*) [55], eucalytus (*Eucalyptus citriodora*) [56]. These species have various activities: insecticidal (Fernande *et al.*, 2002), antibacterial [54, 55] and antifungal [56]. The oxidation of citronellol, a secondary alcohol, produces citronellal [54].

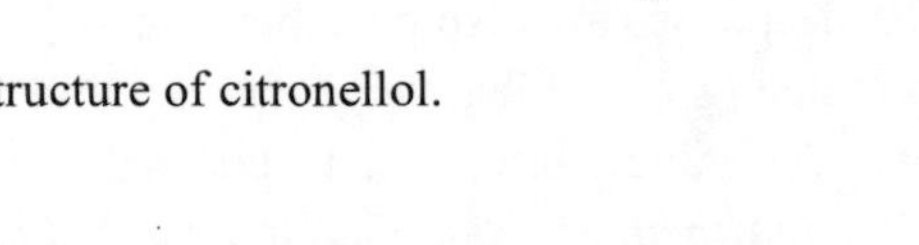

Figure 1. Chemical structure of citronellol.

Citronellal

Citronellal (Fig. 2) is a substance used to make cosmetics and in aromatization of cleaning products, such as soaps and detergents, and because of its antiseptic proprieties, it is used as a cleansing agent, air freshener and disinfectant of floors and bathrooms. The plant *Eucalyptus citriodora* Hook. has been considered the richest source of citronellal and is recognized for its economic importance [57, 58]. Meanwhile, it can also be found as one of the important phytoconstituents of *Cymbopogon citratus* and *Cymbopogon winteranius* [59].

Citronellal can be reduced to make citronellol, which leads to similar line of fragrant substances. L-Menthol can be synthesized from D-citronellal, which is the second most popular fragrance [60].

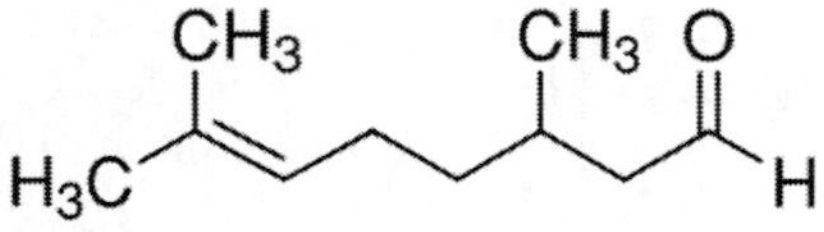

Figure 2. Chemical structure of citronellal.

Myrcene

Among its characteristics, myrcene (Fig. 3) appears as a viscous liquid with a clear yellowish color, possessing a characteristic odor. It has been shown to be a skin and eye irritant, it is inflammable, and its fumes are considered toxic [61].

Myrcene polymerizes when exposed to air and light, resulting in degradation, where temperature is a factor that exerts an influence on its quality [62]. It is part of the composition of oils of various types of herbs. Naturally, it can be found in the oil of laurel, sassafras, verbena and lemongrass, and in the dry flowers of hops and mango of the varieties "cavalo", "rosa", "espada", "palista", "alphonso" and "Jaffna", among other herbs [63, 64] and even in *Cymbopoga citratus* [65] and *Lippia alba,* commonly known as "erva-cidreira" of Northeast Brazil. [66].

In relation to its characteristics, myrcene is an acyclic monoterpene compound, with the chemical name 7-methyl-3-methylene-1,6-octadiene. Various studies have demonstrated its biological activities, where it is able to interfere with the biotransformation of drugs, such as cyclophosphamides, barbiturates and bromobenzene, when present in mammals [67].

Myrcene is considered a noble component, which has been an object of study since 1950, and was evaluated in other bioactivities, such as an intermediate for obtaining of terpene alcohols, chemical fragrances and vitamins A and E [68].

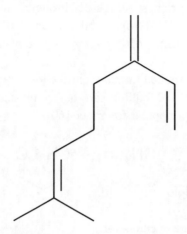

Figure 3. Chemical structure of myrcene.

4. TECHNIQUES OF CONTROL: DIRECT CONTACT AND GASEOUS CONTACT CONTACT DIRECT

Thes techniques start with the determination of the minimal inhibitory concentration (MIC) by the microdilution method using 10% BHI (brain heart infusion) and a bacterial suspension of 10^5 CFU/mL, mixing an initial inoculum of 100 µL with 100 µL of the substance, which was diluted serially giving concentrations of 1024-2 µg/mL [69]. MIC is defined as the lowest concentration at which no microbial growth is observed. MIC of the antibiotics was determined in the presence and absence of the product at a subinhibitory concentration (MIC/8), and the concentrations of antimicrobial drugs used in this assay varied from 1024 to 0.5 µg/mL for the assay. The plates were incubated for 24 h at 37°C [42, 70]. The assay of gaseous contact used five plates by microorganism; in three lids, 100 µL of the product at different concentrations were added, while the two other plates served as a positive and negative control. In the bottom of all the plates, 5 mL of HIA (heart infusion agar) were deposited, which had been seeded with a swab of microorganisms previously grown in BHI (brain heart infusion) for 24 h at 37°C. The method used for antibiotic modulation by gaseous contact was that described by Inouye [71]. The bacterial strains were added to Falcon tubes containing BHI and incubated for 24 h at 37 °C. A sterile swab was immersed in the bacterial suspension, and the bacteria were then seeded on the bottom of plates containing HIA. Three 5-mm disks with different antibiotics were placed on each large plate. The first plate contained the antibiotic disks and the test substance in the lid, while in the second the antibiotic and DMSO in the lid and in third only the antibiotic. The tests were performed in triplicate, where the subinhibitory MID result was used for each bacterial strain.

On all assays performed, were used the standard bacterial strains *K. pneumoniae* ATCC 4362, *S. aureus* ATCC 25923, *P. aerugiosa* 15442 and *E. coli* ATCC 10536, and the multiresistant bacteria *S. aureus* 358 and *E. coli* 27. All strains were donated by the Mycology Laboratory of the Universidade Federal da Paraíba – UFPB.

Antibiotics are substances produced by microorganisms which, at low concentrations, inhibit the growth of other microorganisms. Therefore, the sulfa-type drugs are totally synthetic, for example, and technically are not antibiotics. However, this distinction is often ignored in practice [72]. The antibiotics utilized in this study were aminoglycosides, fluoroquinolones and glycopeptides.

The aminoglycosides are mainly used in the treatment of infections by aerobic Gram-negative bacilli or in synergistic combination with antimicrobial agents that act on the cell wall (e.g., penicillin, ampicillin and vancomycin) against some resistant Gram-positive bacteria, such as enterococci. The members of this group of structurally similar antimicrobial agents inihibit protein synthesis in bacteria at the ribosome level [70]. They bind to the cell surface (cell wall) and then to the bacterial ribosome, impeding the correct reading of messenger RNA and synthesis of the corresponding protein. There are enzymes that inactivate the antibiotic, and these enzymes are coded by genes that are transferred from resistant bacteria to other bacteria through recombination, or plasmid exchange [73, 74]. KNOWLES [75, 76] reports that aminoglycosides enter the cell easily, after altering the permeability of its membrane.

Neomycin is the most toxic antibiotic of the group of aminoglycosides. It is poorly absorbed by the large intestine, and is sometimes administered orally before performing intestinal surgeries, to help control the flora present in the intestine.

Gentamicin is used in the treatment of infections by *P. aeruginosa*, amikacin in infections caused by Gram-negative bacilli and in therapy against mycobacteriosis. Studies on aminoglycosides have revealed that continuous administration of gentamicin causes collateral effects to human health, where it has nephrotoxic potential [77]. It is an antibiotic that interferes with the initial steps of protein synthesis in bacteria, and it is utilized against *Pseudomonas* [72].

Kanamycin and amikacin belong to the class of aminoglycosides derived from the *Streptomyces*. Its bactericidal effect against *M. tuberculosis* is very similar *in vitro* and *in vivo*, where the adverse reactions are the same as those caused by other aminoglycosides. The bactericidal effect of these drugs can be useful in situations of resistance to streptomycin. Cross-resistance between kanamycin and amikacin is common [78].

Vancomycin is part a small group of glycopeptide antibiotics derived from a species of *Streptomyces* found in the jungles of Borneo. Although it has a very small spectrum of activity, which is based on the inhibition of cell wall synthesis, it has been extremely important in dealing with problems due to MRSA [72].

Quinolones are effective agents aganst bacteria, and while they are practically inactive against Gram-positive bacteria, they are still considered very useful in antimicrobial therapy. The can be classified in generations, where the second-generation drugs (norfloxacin and ciprofloxacin) have increased activity against Gram-negative bacteria (including *Pseudomonas aeruginosa*). Ciprofloxacin belongs to the class of antibiotics called fluoroquinolones and is used for treating or preventing certain bacterial infections, where it has wide spectrum of activity [79].

Results and Discussion

According to the results presented in Table 1, citronellol showed antibiotic modulating activity with the bacteria tested, where one of the best results was seen with gentamicin against *S. aureus*, with a significant reduction in its MIC compared to the control.

The essential oil of lemongrass (*Cymbopogon nardus*) a species that presents citronellol showed antibacterial activity against *Listeria monocytogenes*. SCHERER *et al.* [55] showed that palmarosa (*Cymbopogon martinii*), a species that contains citronellol, displayed antibacterial activity against *S. aureus, E. coli* and *Salmonella Thyphimurium*, by means of direct contact. This is the first work on the modulation of antibiotic activity with citronellol, by means of gaseous contact [54].

Table 1. Modulation of aminoglycoside antibiotic activity of citronellol by direct contact

Modulation the Antibiotics of citronellol MIC/8µg/mL				
	E. coli 27		S. aureus 358	
Antibiotics	Alone	Citronellol	Alone	Citronellol
Kanamycin	36,06	39,06	39,06	78,12
Amikacin	156,25	78,12	9,76	78,12
Neomycin	9,76	19,53	19,53	19,53
Gentamicin	39,06	39,06	39,06	9,76

Table 2. Modulation of aminoglycoside antibiotic activity of citronellol by gaseous contact against *Pseudomonas aeruginosa*

Antibiotics	citronellol	Control	DMSO
Ciprofloxacin	2,7cm	2,8cm	2,7cm
Vancomycin	1,6cm	1,5cm	1,7cm
Gentamicin	2,5cm	2,5cm	2,5cm

With regard to the gaseous contact method (Table 2 and 3), the results did not indicate clinically relevant activity, because the size of the inhibition halos for citronellol in combination with antibiotics did not differ much when compared to control, with the largest difference being 0.4 cm for *S. aureus*. DMSO was utilized in testes as the negative control because it was used to dilute the test substances, and thus, this control demonstrated that this solvent did not influence the results.

Table 3. Modulation of aminoglycoside antibiotic activity of citronellol by gaseous contact against *Staphylococcus aureus*

Antibiotics	citronellol	Control	DMSO
Ciprofloxacin	2,3cm	2,3cm	2,2cm
Vancomycin	1,6cm	1,5cm	1,6cm
Gentamicin	1,9cm	2,0cm	1,6cm

Citronellal did not exhibit direct antibacterial activity in the assays, since there was no bacterial growth inhibition at concentrations less than 1024 µg/mL. An analysis of the results for drug-modifying activity revealed that citronellal interacts synergistically with gentamicin enhancing the toxicity of this antibiotic against the strain *E. coli* 27.

A synergistic effect was also demonstrated when citronellal was combined with amikacin and neomycin in the assays against *S.aureus* 358. Meanwhile, an antagonistic effect was seen when this compound was combined with the aminoglycoside kanamycin (Table 4). In the gaseous contact assays, citronellal inhibited the growth of *P. aeruginosa*, but not at a clinically relevant concentration (Table 5 and 6), considering that the difference in the size of the inhibition halos was small when comparing citronellal to the control.

Table 4. Modulation of aminoglycoside antibiotic activity of citronellal by direct contact

Modulation the Antibiotics of citronellal MIC/8µg/mL				
	E. coli 27		*S. aureus* 358	
Antibiotics	alone	citronellal	Alone	citronellal
Kanamycin	39,06	39,06	156,25	39,06
Amikacin	9,76	9,76	39,06	156,25
Neomycin	19,53	19,53	2,44	9,76
Gentamicin	4,88	39,06	39,06	39,06

Table 5. Modulation of aminoglycoside antibiotic activity of citronellal by gaseous contact against *Pseudomonas aeruginosa*

Antibiotics	citronellal	Control	DMSO
Ciprofloxacin	3,0cm	3,0cm	3,0cm
Vancomycin	1,8cm	2,8cm	1,8cm
Gentamicin	2,1cm	2,3cm	2,0cm

Table 6. Modulation of aminoglycoside antibiotic activity of citronellal by gaseous contact against *Staphylococcus aureus*

Antibiotics	citronellal	Control	DMSO
Ciprofloxacin	2,7cm	2,6cm	2,6cm
Vancomycin	1,8cm	1,8cm	1,8cm
Gentamicin	2,3cm	2,8cm	2,2cm

Table 7. Modulation of aminoglycoside antibiotic activity
of myrcene by direct contact

Modulation the Antibiotics of myrcene CIM/8µg/ml				
	E. coli 27		*S. aureus* 358	
Antibiotics	Alone	myrcene	alone	myrcene
Kanamycin	78,12	19,53	19,53	19,53
Amikacin	78,12	39,06	78,12	78,12
Neomycin	78,12	19,53	9,76	39,06
Gentamicin	39,06	39,06	4,88	4,88

The combination of antibiotics can cause different effects, one of them being antagonism. Antagonistic effects have been reported for the combination of different antibiotics and of antibiotics with natural products. Such effect has been attributed to the mutual chelation of drugs [80, 81]. Such an effect may have occured with the combination of citronellal and kanamycin.

Previous studies have confirmed that a natural product can potentiate the action of another natural product, whether of animal or plant origin, demonstrating that the interaction of the drugs can indicate a new path for the formulation of drugs in combination [5, 42, 44, 82].

In the determination of the minimal inhibitory concentration of myrcene, the results demonstrated that myrcene does not possess clinically relevant antibacterial activity, showing a MIC $\geq$1024µg/mL. An antagonistic effect was found when myrcene was combined with neomycin and tested against *S. aureus* 358. However, an interesting synergism was demonstrated when combining myrcene with kanamycin and neomycin against the Gram-negative bacteria *E. coli* 27, providing evidence that myrcene potentiated the action of the antibiotics (Table 7).

In assays using gaseous contact, myrcene did not show antibacterial activity at the doses tested against any of the microorganisms used. Its combination with the antibiotics vancomycin, ciprofloxacin and gentamicin showed no difference, where there was no enhancement of the effect of the drugs, considering that the majority of the inhibition zones were greater than in the control in the absence of the oil compound (Table 8 and 9).

Myrcene has already been investigated with respect to its fungitoxic activity against phytopathogens, but its inhibitory effect on mycelia growth was zero against all the fungi tested [83].

Table 8. Modulatory of aminoglycoside antibiotic activity by gaseous contact against *Pseudomonas aeruginosa* by Myrcene

Antibiotics	myrcene	Control	DMSO
Ciprofloxacin	1,7cm	1,7cm	1,7cm
Vancomycin	2,7cm	2,5cm	2,7cm
Gentamicin	2,3cm	2,3cm	2,0cm

Table 9. Modulatory of aminoglycoside antibiotic activity by gaseous contact against *Staphylococcus aureus* by Myrcene

Antibióticos	myrcene	Control	DMSO
Ciprofloxacin	1,7cm	1,7cm	1,7cm
Vancomycin	2,5cm	1,8cm	2,5cm
Gentamicin	2,9cm	2,8cm	2,2cm

The essential oil of lemongrass (*Cymbopoga citratus* DC Stapf) is composed of myrcene, neral and geranial, and its antimicrobial action was reported by NGUEFACK [84]. However, the results of these works do not indicate myrcene as being responsible for such activity, since myrcene was not tested alone, and thus, this activity can be attributed to other phytoconstituents or even to their combination.

CONCLUSION AND PERSPECTIVE

The utilization of medicinal plants goes back to ancient times; however, there is still a great need for advancements in research nowadays. The development of studies along this line, regardless of the scientific viewpoint, is part of the domain of molecular bioprospecting.

Molecular bioprospecting along with the study of natural products will have a special role in the future, because in a multidisciplinary way, it aims to obtain information about the applicability of chemical substances from biological material for various purposes, and at the same time emphasizing the importance of its sustainable use.

The search for more effective active principles that are less harmful to humans has given research on medicinal plants in a distinquished place in our scientific scope and has thus created new perspectives for studies in ethnopharmacology, phytochemistry and microbiology, among others.

[21] Georgopapadakou, NH; Liu, FY. Penicillin-binding proteins in bacteria. Antimicrob. *Agents Chemother*, 1980, v. 18, p. 148-157.

[22] Neves, MC; Rossi, ODJ; Alves, ECC; Lemos, MVF. Detecção de genes de resistência antimicrobiana em cromossomos e plasmídeos de *Staphylococcus spp*. Arquivo Instituto Biológico, 2007, v. 74, n. 3, p. 207-213.

[23] Carvalho, WA. Quinolonas. In: Silva, P. "Farmacologia". Guanabara Koogan. Rio de Janeiro, 1998.

[24] Korolkovas, A; Lopez, MLL; Marangoni, AN. Fluorquinolonas: Gênese, Mecanismo de Ação e Uso Terapêutico. Revista Brasileira de Medicina, 1992, v. 49, n. 6, p. 267-284.

[25] Campbell.-J.r., GD; Silberman, R. Drug-resistant Streptococcus pneumoniae. *Clinical Infectious Disease,* 1998, v. 26, p. 1188-1195.

[26] Schreiber, JR; Jacobs, MR. Pneumococos resistentes a antibióticos. In: Schreiber, JR.; Goldman, DA. "Clínicas Pediátricas da América do Norte". Interlivros, Rio de Janeiro, 1995.

[27] Smith, JT; Amyes, SGB. Bacterial resistance to Antifolate Chemotherapeutic Agents Mediated by Plasmids. *British Medical Bulletin*, 1984, v. 40, n. 1, p. 42-46.

[28] Livermore, DM. Bacterial resistance: origins, epidemiology, and impact. *Clinical Infectious Disease,* 2003, v. 36, p. 11-23.

[29] Silveira, GP; Nome, F; Gesser, JC; Sá, MM. Estratégias utilizadas no combate a resistência bacteriana. *Quimica Nova*, 2006, v. 29, n. 4, p. 844-855.

[30] Piddock, LJV. Clinically relevant chromosomally encoded multidrug resistance efflux pumps in bacterial. *Journal Clinical Microbiology,* 2006, v. 19, p. 382-402.

[31] Silva, MB; Nicoli, Λ; Costa, ASV; Brasileiro BG; Jamal CM; Silva CA; Paula Junior, TJ; Texeira H. Ação antimicrobiana de extratos de plantas medicinais sobre espécies fitopatogênicas de fungos do gênero Colletotrichum. *Revista Brasileira de Plantas Medicinais*, 2008, v. 10, n. 3, p. 57-60.

[32] Salvagnini, LE; Oliveira, JRS; Santos, LE; Moreira, RRD; Pietro, RCLR. Evaluation ofthe antibacterial activity of Myrtus communis L. (Myrtaceae) leaves. *Revista Brasileira de Farmacognosia*, 2008, v. 18, p. 241–244.

[33] Simões, CC; Araujo, DB; Araújo, RPC. Study, in vitro and ex vivo, of the action of different concentrations of propolis extracts against

microorganisms present in human saliva. *Revista Brasileira de Farmacognosia*, 2008, v. 18, p. 84–89.

[34]   Gibbons S. Anti-staphylococcal plant natural products. *Natural Product Reports*, 2004, v. 21, p. 263-277.

[35]   Gurib – Fakim, A. Medicinal plants: Traditions of yesterday and drugs of tomorrouw. *Molecular Aspects of Medicine*, 2006, v. 27, p. 91-93.

[36]   Daferera, DJ; Ziogas, BN; Polissiou, MG. The effectiveness of plant essential oils on the growth of Botrytis cinerea, Fusarium sp. and Clavibacter michiganesis subsp. Michiganesis. *Crop Protection*, 2003, v. 22, p. 39-44.

[37]   Nicolson, K; Evans, G; O'Toole, PW. Potentiation of methicillin activity againstmethicillin-resistant *Staphylococcus aureus* by diterpenes. *FEMS Microbiology Letters,* 1999, v. 179, p. 233–239.

[38]   Burt, S. Essential oils: their antibacterial properties and potential applicationsin foods – a review. *International Journal Food Microbiology*,2004, v. 94, p. 223–53.

[39]   Wendakoon, C; Sakaguchi, M. Inhibition of amino acid decarboxylase activity of *Enterobacter aerogenes* by active components in spices. *Journal of Food Protection*, 1995, v. 58, p. 280–283.

[40]   Coutinho, HDM; Costa, JG; Lima, EO; Falcão-Silva, VS; Siqueira-Júnior, JP. Enhancement of the antibiotic activity against a multiresistant *Escherichia coli* by *Mentha arvensis* L. and chlorpromazine. *Chemotherapy*, 2008, 54, 328-330.

[41]   Coutinho, HDM; Costa JGM; Lima, EO; Falcão-Silva, VS; Siqueira-Jr, JP. In vitro interference of Hyptis martiusii Benth. & chlorpromazine against an aminoglycoside - resistant *Escherichia coli*. *Indian Journal Medical Residency*, v. 2009b, v. 129, p. 566-568.

[42]   42 Coutinho, HDM; Costa, JGM; Falcão-Silva, VS; Siqueira-Júnior, JP; Lima, EO. *In vitro* additive effect of *Hyptis martiusii* in the resistance to aminoglycosides of methicillin-resistant *Staphylococcus aureus*. *Pharmaceutical Biology*, 2010, v. 48, n. 9, p. 1002–1006.

[43]   Wagner, H; Ulrich-Merzenich, G. Synergy research: approaching a new gener ation of phytopharmaceuticals. *Phytomedicine*, 2009, v. 16, p. 97–110.

[44]   Coutinho, HDM; Costa, JGM; Lima, EO; Falcão-Silva, VS; Siqueira-JR, JP. Increasing of the Aminoglicosyde Antibiotic Activity Against a Multidrug-Resistant *E. coli* by *Turnera ulmifolia* L. and Chlorpromazine. *Biological Ressearch for Nursing*, 2010b, v. 11, p. 332.

[45] Cunha, FAB; Matias, EFF; Brito, SV; Ferreira, FS; Braga JMA; Costa, JGM; Coutinho, HDM. Phytochemical screening, antibacterial activity and in vitro interactions between Costus cf. arabicus L. with UV-A and aminoglycosides. *Natural Product Research*, 2011, v. 26, n. 4, p. 380-386.

[46] Matias, *EF; Santos, KK; Almeida, TS; Costa, JG; Coutinho, HD*M. Atividade antibacteriana In vitro de Croton campestris A., Ocimum gratissimum L. e Cordia verbenacea DC. Revista Brasileira de Biociências, 2010, v. 8, n.3, p.294-298.

[47] Siqui, AC; Sampaio, ALF; Sousa, MC; Henriques, MGMO; Ramos, MFS. Óleos essenciais - potencial antiinflamatório. *Biotecnologia: Ciência e Desenvolvimento*, 2000, v. 16, p. 38-43.

[48] Wink, M. Phisiology of secondary product formation in plants. In Charlwood, BV. and Rhodes, MJC. "Secondary products from plant tissue culture". Clarendon, Oxford, 1990.

[49] Harborne, JB. "Introduction to ecological biochemistry." Academic, London, 1988.

[50] Deans, SG; Waterman, PG. Biological Activity of Volatile Oils. In: Hay, RKM. and Waterman, GP. (Ed). "Volatile oil crops: their biology, biochemistry and production." John Willey & Sons. Londres, 1993.

[51] Adam, K; Sivropoulou, A; Kokkini, S; Lanaras, T; Arsenakis, M. Antifungal activities of *Origanum vulgare* subsp. *Hirtun, Mentha spicata, Lavandula angustifolia* and *Salvia fruticosa* essencial oils human pathogenic fungi. *Journal of Agricultural and Food Chemistry*, 1998, v. 46, p. 1739-1745.

[52] Hulin, V; Mathot, A.-G; Mafart, P; Dufosse, L. Les proprieties anti-microbiennes des huiles essentielles te composes d'arômes. *Sciences des aliments*, 1998, v. 18, p.563-582.

[53] Mattos, SH. "Estudos Fitotécnicos da *Mentha arvensis* L. var. Holmes como produtora de mentol no Ceará." PhD Thesis – Universidade Federal do Ceará, Fortaleza, 2000.

[54] Oliveira, MMM; Brugnera, DF; Cardoso, MG; Guimarães, LGL; Piccoli, RH. Rendimento, composição química e atividade antilisterial de óleos essenciais de espécies de *Cymbopogon*. *Revista Brasileira de Plantas Medinais*, 2011, v. 13, n. 1, p. 8-16.

[55] Scherer, R; Wagner, R; Duarte, MCT; Godoy, HT. Composição e atividades antioxidante e antimicrobiana dos óleos essenciais de cravo-da-índia, citronela e palmarosa. *Revista Brasileira de Plantas Medinais*, 2009, v. 11, n. 4, p. 442-449.

[56] Bonaldo, SM; Schwan-Estrada, KF; Stangarlin, JR; Tessmann, DJ; Scapim, CA. Fungitoxicidade, Atividade Elicitora de Fitoalexinas e Proteção de Pepino contra *Colletotrichum lagenarium*, pelo Extrato Aquoso de *Eucalyptus citriodora*. *Revista Fitopatologia Brasileira*, 2004, v. 29, n. 2, p. 128-134.

[57] Vitti, AMS. "Avaliação do crescimento e do rendimento e qualidade do óleo essencial de rocedências de *Eucalyptus citriodora*." MSc. Thesis - Escola Superior Luiz de Queiroz, Piracicaba, 1999, p. 83.

[58] Matos, FJA. "Farmácias vivas: sistema de utilização de plantas medicinais projetado para pequenas comunidades." Editora UFC, Fortaleza, 2002.

[59] Pereira, FO. "Atividade antifúngica do óleo essencial de *Cymbopogom winterianus* Jowitt ex Bor sobre dermatófitos do gênero *Trichophyton*." MSc. Thesis - Universidade Federal da Paraíba - UFPB, João Pessoa, 2009.

[60] Craveiro, AA; Queiroz, DC. "Óleos essenciais e química fina." Editora UFC. Fortaleza, 1992.

[61] Kolicheski, MB. "Síntese do Mirceno a partir da isomerização térmica do β-pipeno." PhD Thesis - Universidade Federal do Paraná, Curitiba, 2006.

[62] Virmani, OP; Srivastava, R; Datta, SG. "*Oil of lemongrass*." Part 2: West Indian, World Crops, 1979.

[63] Andrade, EHA; Maia, JGS; Zoghbi, MGB. Aroma volatile constituents of brazilian varieties of mango fruit. *Journal of Food Composition and Analysis*, 2000, v. 13, p. 27-33.

[64] Merck. "*The Merck Index - Encyclopedia of Chemicals, Drugs and Biologicals*." Merck and CO. NJ, [USA], 1989.

[65] Craveiro, AA; Fernandes, AG; Andrade, CHS; Matos, FJA; Alencar, JW; Machado, MIL. "*Óleos essenciais de plantas do nordeste*." Editora UFC, Fortaleza, 1981.

[66] Matos, FJA. As ervas cidreiras do nordeste do Brasil. Estudo de três quimiotipos de *Lippia alba* (Mill). N.E.Br- Verbenaceae. *Revista Brasileira de Farmacognosia*, 1996, v. 77, p. 137-141.

[67] Oliveira, ACAX; Pinto, LFR; Paumgartten, FJR. In vitro inhibition of CYP2B1 monooxygenase by β-myrcene and other monoterpenoid compounds. *Toxicology Letters*, 1997, v. 92, p. 39-46.

[68] Kirk, RE; Othmer, DF. "*Encyclopedia of Chemical Technology*." John Wiley and Sons. New York, 1981.

[69] Javadepour, MM; Juban, MM; LO, WC; Bishop, SM; Alberty, JB; Mann, CM; Markhan, J.L. A new method for determine the minimum inhibitory concentration of essential oils. *Journal of Applied Microbiology*, 1998, v. 84, p. 538–544.

[70] NCCLS. "Methods for Dilution Antimicrobial Susceptibility Tests for Bacteria That Grow Aerobically". *Approved Standard—Sixth Edition.* NCCLS document M7-A6 [ISBN 1-56238-486-4]. NCCLS, 940 West Valley Road, Suite 1400, Wayne, Pennsylvania 19087-1898 USA, 2003.

[71] Inouye, S; Takizawa, T; Yamaguchi, H. Antibacterial activity of essential oils and their major constituents against respiratory tract pathogens by gaseous contact. *Journal of Antimicrobial Chemotherapy*, 2001, v. 47, p. 565-573.

[72] Tortora, GJ; Funke, BR; Case, CL. "Microbiologia." Artmed, Porto Alegre, 2008.

[73] Barbosa, FHF; *Silva, AM; Duarte, R; Nicoli, JR.* Perfil de susceptibilidade antimicrobiana de *Bifidobacterium bifidum* Bb12 e *Bifidumbacterium longun* Bb46. Revista de Biologia e Ciências da Terra, 2001, v. 1, n. 2, p. 345-349.

[74] Tavares, W. "Manual de antibioticos e quimioterápicos anti-infecciosos." Atheneu, São Paulo, 1996.

[75] Knowles, JR; Roller, S; Murray, DB; Naidu, AS. Antimicrobial action of carvacol at different stages of dual-species biofilm development by staphylococcus aureus and salmonella ty phimurium. *Applied and Environmental Microbiology*, 2005, v. 71, n. 2, p. 797-803.

[76] Pelczar Jr, MJ. "Microbiologia conceitos e aplicações." *Makron Books*, São Paulo, 1997.

[77] Giacoia, GP; Shentag, JJ. Pharmacokinetics and nephrotoxicity of continuous infusion of gentamicin in low birth weight infants. *Journal of Pediatrics*, 1986, v. 109, p.715-719.

[78] World Health Organization Treatment of tuberculosis: guidelines for national programmes. Report nuber WHO/CDS/TB, 2003, p. 313.

[79] Olivares, ATS; Vidal, VV. Uso y abuso del ciprofloxacino. Medisan, 2011, v. 15, n. 3, p. 384-392.

[80] Granowitz, EV; Brown, RB. Antibiotic adverse reactions and drug interactions. *Critical Care Clinics*, 2008, v. 24, p. 421–442.

[81] Ferreira, SF; Brito, SV; Costa, JG; Alves, RR; Coutinho, HD; Almeida, WO. Is the body fat of the lizard *Tupinambis merianae* effective against bacterial infections? *Journal of Ethnopharmacology*, 2009, v. 126, p. 233–237.

[82] Coutinho, HDM; Costa, JGM; Lima, EO; Siqueira-Jr, JP. Additive effects of *Hyptis martiusii* Benth with aminoglycosides against *Escherichia coli*. *Indian Journal of Medical Research*, 2010, v. 131, p. 106-108.

[83] Guimarães, LGL; Cardoso, MG; Paulo, SE; Andrade, J; Vieira, SS., Atividades antioxidante e fungitóxica do óleo essencial de capim-limão e do citral. *Revista Ciência Agronômicas*, 2011, v. 42, n. 2, p. 464-472.

[84] Nguefack, J; Budde, BB; Jakobsen, M. Five essential oils from aromatic plants of Cameroon: their antibacterial activity and ability to permeabilize the cytoplasmic membrane of *Listeria innocua* examined by flow cytometry. *Letters in Applied Microbiology*, 2004, v. 39, n. 5, p. 395-400.

In: Gentamicin
Editor: Emilie Kruger

ISBN: 978-1-62808-841-0
© 2013 Nova Science Publishers, Inc.

Chapter 4

REGIOSPECIFIC GENTAMICIN FUNCTIONALIZATION: DESIGN FOR PARTICULAR APPLICATIONS

Jonathan Grote[*], *Richard Himmelsbach* and *Don Johnson*

Organic Chemistry Process Research,
Abbott Diagnostics Division, IL, US

ABSTRACT

Gentamicin is an aminoglycoside antibiotic naturally synthesized by *Micromonospora*, a Gram-positive genus of bacteria widely found in water and soil. This antibiotic is useful against a wide variety of bacteria, and works by binding the 30S subunit of the bacterial ribosome, which interrupts bacterial protein synthesis. High serum concentrations of gentamicin can result in permanent damage to the balance and orientation components of the inner ear, and can have nephrotoxic effects in renal cells, potentially leading to renal failure.

Gentamicin is a complex consisting of several structurally different components. The three major constituents the gentamicin complex, C1, C2, and C1a, differ only by the presence or absence of methyl groups in different locations on each molecule, the relative proportions of which can vary widely depending on how the antibiotic was cultured or isolated.

---

[*] Corresponding author's email: jon.grote@abbott.com.

Each component has five different amino groups and three hydroxyl groups, and contains two acid sensitive glycosidic linkages. The presence of these multiple reactive groups in each component present considerable challenges to selective modification of gentamicin.

It would thus be useful to be able to regiospecifically functionalize gentamicin in order to tailor the derivatization to meet the needs of a particular application. This paper will describe a variety of methods that have proven useful for the regiospecific functionalization of gentamicin at different locations.

Gentamicin is an aminoglycoside complex naturally synthesized by *Micromonospora*, a Gram-positive genus of bacteria commonly present in water and soil [1]. This antibiotic is active against several different types of bacteria, functioning by binding the 30S subunit of the bacterial ribosome, which interrupts bacterial protein synthesis. [2]

Gentamicin is not usually administered orally, due to the potential for degradation in the digestive tract, but instead is given intravenously, intramuscularly, or topically to treat bacterial infections. [3] Serum concentrations of gentamicin should be carefully monitored, since overdoses can result in permanent damage to the balance and orientation components of the inner ear, as well as nephrotoxic effects in renal cells, which can potentially lead to renal failure. [4]

C1: $R_1 = R_2 = CH_3$
C2, C2a: $R_1 = CH_3$, $R_2 = H$
C1a: $R_1 = R_2 = H$

The gentamicin complex is commercially manufactured by fermentation, and typically consists of three major components C1, C1a, and C2, as well as several minor constituents. Specifically, the structure of gentamicin's major components consists of a middle 2-deoxystreptamine moiety (C1-C6) glycosidically linked to two other saccharide units, a purpurosamine on the northern end (C1'-C6') and a garosamine on the southern end (C1"-C5") as shown. The structures of these three components differ only by the presence or absence of methyl groups in two different locations on the purpurosamine of each molecule, [5] the relative proportions of which can vary widely depending on what conditions were used to culture or isolate the antibiotic. Careful examination of the chemical structure of these components reveals numerous different types and chemical environments of amino and hydroxyl groups in each component, which would be expected to react unselectively to produce a complex mixture during chemical modification reactions. The glycosidic linkages present in each molecule also preclude the use of strongly acidic reagents during organic transformations. The lack of UV active functionality presents an additional challenge for monitoring the progress of gentamicin functionalization.

Non-selective conjugation of gentamicin has been frequently utilized in numerous situations, and has provided satisfactory results for a number of applications, including the determination of the presence of gentamicin, the relative ratio of the three components, or the absence of one of the three components. Each method typically imparts a moiety that is detectable by the analytical method. Three groups have reported non-specific derivitization of gentamicin with 9-fluorenylmethyl chloroformate (FMOC-Cl), useful for detection during HPLC analysis employing fluorescence detection. [6, 7] Chen and co-workers further developed an ELISA by treatment of a mixture of gentamicin components and bovine serum albumin or ovalbumin with glutaraldehyde followed by sodium borohydride, or by conjugating gentamicin components to either protein with EDAC. [8] Jin and co-workers similarly non-specifically conjugated gentamicin to keyhole limpet hemocyanin and horse radish peroxidase in their successful development of a competitive direct ELISA for gentamicin. [9] Gentamicin BSA conjugates have been used to prepare colloidal gold constructs to probe the precise biochemical events leading to bactericidal activity. [10] Non-selective Texas Red conjugates of gentamicin have been prepared by Schmid and co-workers by reaction of Texas Red succinimidyl active ester with gentamicin sulfate in DMF, with the aim of identifying the target cells in the inner ear of the rat by using short-time exposure and low-dose application of gentamicin with fluorescence microscopy. [11] Gentamicin has also been non-specifically conjugated to agarose beads, enabling development of a gentamicin-agarose pull-down assay useful for isolating gentamicin-binding proteins (GBPs) from cells. [12]

However, given the chemical complexity of gentamicin, it would be useful to regiospecifically functionalize gentamicin in order to tailor the modification to meet the needs of a particular application. Theoretically, two strategies could be useful to achieve these needs. One option would be to develop a regioselective reagent or method which would be insensitive to the variety of environments found for the different hydroxyl or amino groups present in the three components. Since both of the structural variations (the presence or absence of the two methyl groups) occur in the purpurosamine ring of the three components, this reagent or method would likely operate on one of the two lower rings, which are identical for all three components. This strategy would be advantageous, in that no material would be discarded, since all three components would be utilized. Analysis of the chemical reactions could be challenging, however, since the reactions would be complex, due to the need to simultaneously monitor any modification of all three different components simultaneously.

A different strategy would be to first separate the components, and regioselectively chemically modify one of the separated components. The advantages of this strategy are that the number of components is reduced, substantially reducing the number of chemical environments present and theoretically enabling the reaction to proceed regiospecifically, or allowing the use of a less regioselective reagent to obtain satisfactory modification results. This strategy is advantageous, in that reaction monitoring would be straightforward due to the presence of one reactant and one product. However, it is disadvantageous in that two components (potentially two-thirds of the material depending on culture production) of the starting gentamicin complex would not be utilized after separation.

In practice, use of either strategy has been employed, depending on the ultimate use of the derivitized product. Protecting groups can be used to enhance the success of either strategy. By regioselectively protecting some of the more reactive amino or hydroxyl groups, less reactive groups can be selectively functionalized. Deprotection provides the regiospecifically derivatized gentamicin.

Examination of prior work indicates that the large scale separation of the three major components of the gentamicin complex is challenging and labor intensive. [13] Chromatographic systems, by necessity, must employ polar, protic solvents such as alcohols and ammonia to elute the three components off of a solid phase. Trial and error elution profiles are required to obtain enough acceptably pure fractions. If underivatized, the separated fractions of gentamicin must be visualized, which is straightforward if analyzed by thin layer chromatography.

The final isolated product is difficult to characterize by microanalysis due to solvent inclusion, not unexpected with the many polar amino and hydroxyl groups that gentamicin possesses. [14, 15] Repeated attempts to isolate pure materials are further challenged due to the tendency of gentamicin free bases to be hygrospopic.

Due to these limitations, we sought a methodology that allowed for the separation of the three major components of gentamicin and simultaneously provided the purified materials in a characterizable form. HPLC would be an ideal methodology for separating large amounts of the three components of the gentamicin complex, and UV is a commonly used method for detection. However, gentamicin components would need to be modified to be detectable. Protection of the hydroxyl or amino groups of gentamicin with a UV active protecting group would render gentamicin transiently detectable, and removal of the protecting groups after separation under mild conditions would provide the individual gentamicin free bases. Several attempts to use a variety of well-known protecting groups to produce good yields of regioselectively protected gentamicin proved to be challenging in our hands, due to the production of a plethora of products from these reactions as previously noted. Both hydroxyl and amine protection strategies were demonstrated to be untenable.

Upon further consideration, we theorized that protection of *all* reactive groups in gentamicin might be the best way to obtain high yields of single products. Separation of the fully protected products could then theoretically be achieved by HPLC. While there are fewer hydroxyl groups (three) than amino groups (five) present in the three components of gentamicin, unprotected amino groups are more polar and tend to render molecules hydroscopic and make them less easily handled than unprotected hydroxyl groups. We thus decided that amino group protection would be a better option. Among UV active amine protecting groups, the FMOC and CBz protecting groups emerged as ideal choices because they can be introduced under basic conditions, avoiding the use of acidic reagents which could potentially degrade the glycosidic linkages present in gentamicin components. Since the FMOC group is typically removed by reaction with volatile, low molecular weight amines, but produces 9-fluorenylmethanol as a side product, which would necessitate purification, CBz was selected as the preferred group, since it can be cleaved using catalytic hydrogenation and produces a volatile side product (toluene), allowing for straightforward isolation of the pure deprotected products simply by catalyst filtration and evaporation.

Small scale protection of the gentamicin complex with multiple equivalents of benzyl chloroformate using Shotten-Baumen conditions employing sodium carbonate resulted in full protection of all five amino groups and straightforward isolation after an ethyl acetate – water workup. This reaction was easily scaled up to provide multiple grams of protected material suitable for subsequent HPLC purification. With fully protected material in hand, we sought a combination of an HPLC solid phase and mobile phase which would provide a satisfactory separation of the three protected components. After screening a number of different combinations of solid phase and mobile aqueous phase with different aqueous modifiers, we were gratified to find that elution of the YMC ODS-AQ solid support with aqueous ammonium formate/acetonitrile mixtures provided good separation of the three protected components. [16] Ammonium formate was an ideal choice of aqueous modifier, because it permitted good resolution of the three components and was fully removed during the lyophilization process. This permitted a straightforward isolation of the fully protected gentamicin components by lyophilization, to produce white solids that were easily handled, fully soluble in organic solvents, and provided satisfactory analytical data due to the lack of the presence of occluded solvents. [14] Furthermore, commercial availability of both analytical and preparative YMC ODS-AQ columns facilitated testing of the separation process with different eluents, analysis of the separated fractions, and scaling up of the isomer separation process. Component purities of 95.9-99.2% by analytical HPLC and overall mass recoveries of 60-70% could be obtained in one pass by careful fraction collection, with the balance of material recoverable for resubmission to the separation process.

Once the three protected components were separated, analysis by electrospray mass spectrometry, commonly used to identify gentamicin and its degradation products, was employed to determine the identity of the three components. We were pleased that the material from the first peak showed (M + NH$_4$)$^+$ at 1138.7, correlating well with the calculated molecular mass of protected gentamicin C1a of 1120.2. The material from each of the second and third peaks (partially resolved) showed the same mass spectral data [(M + NH$_4$)$^+$ at 1152.3], both correlating to the molecular mass of protected gentamicin C2 and C2a at 1134.2. Material from the last peak was confirmed as gentamcicin C1, having (M + NH$_4$)$^+$ at 1166.4, which correlated well with the molecular mass of protected gentamicin C1 at 1148.3 (see Figure 1 below).

Further corroboration of the identities of the three separated components was obtained after deprotection, which was achieved in quantitative yield under atmospheric pressure catalytic hydrogenation conditions. Straightforward workup (catalyst filtration and concentration) provided the three purified components as amorphous white solids. The C1a component after deprotection showed $(M + H)^+$ at 450.3 and $(2M + H)^+$ at 900.0., consistent with a molecular mass of 449.5. The deprotected C2/C2a components showed $(M + H)^+$ at 464.3 and $(2M + H)^+$ at 928.0, consistent with a molecular mass of 463.6, and the deprotected C1 component showed $(M + H)^+$ at 478.3 and $(2M + H)^+$ at 956.1, consistent with a molecular mass of 477.6 (Figure 1 below).

As demonstrated above, this methodology, including protection of the gentamicin complex with benzyl chloroformate, separation of the protected components by HPLC with UV detection, and deprotection of the separated protected isomers, provides a simple yet elegant method for the large scale separation of the three components of the gentamicin complex. [16] Both the protected and deprotected components are isolated in pure form and readily reactive in subsequent steps.

Gentamicin C1 is the component that has the least number of primary amino groups, and has thus been chosen for use in the design of new derivatives prepared by regioselective N-acylation by several researchers. For example, Daniels and co-workers published a study which sought to improve gentamicin's antibiotic activity, particularly against gentamicin resistant organisms. [17]

This group started with gentamicin C1. Reaction of C1 with one equivalent of ethyl trifluorothiolactate followed by chromatography provided 2'-N-trifluoroacetylgentamicin C1 **1** (69% yield; Figure 2).

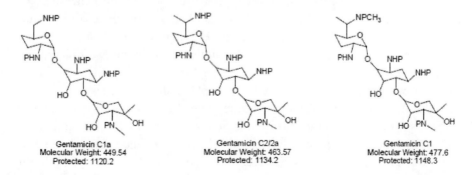

Gentamicin C1a
Molecular Weight: 449.54
Protected: 1120.2

Gentamicin C2/2a
Molecular Weight: 463.57
Protected: 1134.2

Gentamicin C1
Molecular Weight: 477.6
Protected: 1148.3

Figure 1. Structures and masses of individual gentamicin complex components in elution order (P = CBz).

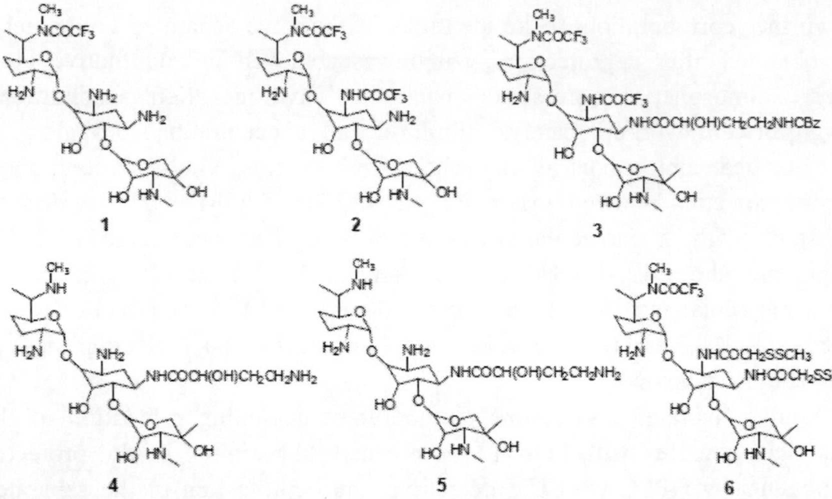

Figure 2. Regioselective aminohydroxybutyl, aminohydroxypropyl, and diacylated gentamicin derivatives.

Treatment of **2** with one additional equivalent of ethyl trifluorothiolactate produced 2',3-di-N-trifluoroacetylgentamicin C1 **2** (42% yield after chromatography). Two equivalents of ethyl trifluoroacetyl thiolactate produced also produced **2** (34% yield). This indicated that the 2'-amino group in gentamicin C1 showed the highest reactivity, followed by the 3-amino group. Subsequent reaction of **2** with 1.2 equivalents of N-[(S)-4-benzyl-oxycarbonylamino-2-hydroxybutyroxy]succinimide produced **3** (51% yield), which when deprotected provided 1-N-[(S)-4-amino-2-hydroxy-butyl] gentamicin **4** in 78% yield after chromatography. 1-N-[(S)-3-amino-2-hydroxypropyl]gentamicin **5** was also prepared in a similar manner.

Singh and co-workers reacted the 2'-N-trifluoroacetylated gentamicin C1 **1** described above with methyldithioacetic acid (EDAC mediated) to produce 1,3- bis(methyldithioacetyl)-2'-N-trifluoroacetyl gentamicin C1 **6** (20% yield, latter fractions, Figure 2, above). [18] Reduction cleaved the two dithianes, to produce a dithiogentamicin derivative which was conjugated in its trifluoroacetylated form to glucose-6-phosphate dehydrogenase which had been functionalized via bromoacetylation. The gentamicin-enzyme conjugate was used to develop a homogeneous enzyme immunoassay for gentamicin.

Wright received a patent describing the selective functionalization of the 1-position gentamicins as well as other aminoglycoside antibiotics. [19] In this case, regioselective functionalization was achieved by reacting protected aminoglycosides with free 3"- and 1-amino groups with a variety of Nalkyloxycarbonylimidazoles. A high yielding regioselective protection reaction occurs at the 3"-amino group under these conditions, allowing for subsequent regioselective functionalization at the 1-position, to produce a family of antibiotics with high potency after deprotection.

Additionally, Litovchick and co-workers conjugated arginine to the gentamicin complex, to produce primarily two conjugates. [20] While not a strictly regioselective reaction, the primary products obtained confirm the results above. The gentamicin C1/C2 tri-arginine product ("R3G") was the primary functionalization product, resulting from reaction of the C1 and C2 gentamicin components at the 1, 2', and 3-amino groups as expected in light of Daniels and co-workers observations (vide supra). A gentamicin C1a tetra-arginine conjugate was also produced, by reaction of gentamicin C1a at the 6'-amino group (a primary amine in gentamicin C1a) in addition to the other three reactive amino groups. The conjugates, after labeling with fluorescein isothiocyanate, inhibited interactions between compositions of bacterial RNase P (PRNA) and protein [21] and as Tat antagonists [22] with the aim of targeting HIV by inhibiting replication.

In an interesting non-traditional modification of the reactivity observed above, several researchers have described studies employing *complexation* of gentamicin as a method for selective functionalization. With its large number of unsubstituted amino and hydroxyl groups, gentamicin as well as other aminoglycoside antibiotics are natural targets for testing the ability of multivalent metals, especially transition metals, to regioselectively complex amino groups and render them unreactive toward protection reagents, effectively making them transitory protecting groups.

Nagabushan and co-workers first described the amine protection of transition metal complexed aminoglycoside antibiotics. [23] They found that divalent transition metal cations selectively complexed pairs of amino and hydroxyl groups, which effectively prevented conventional protecting groups from reacting at these groups.

Specifically, separated gentamicin components C1, C2, or C1a were first complexed with $Ni^{2}+$ or Cu^{2+} in polar aprotic solvents to form the complex **7** (vide infra), and subsequently reacted at the uncomplexed amino groups with protecting reagents such as N-(benzyloxycarbonyl)phthalimide and N-(trichloroethoxycarbonyloxy) succinimide to provide the 2',3,6'-tri-N-protected aminoglycosides. In this way, high yields of triprotected glycosides were prepared, enabling subsequent regioselective chemical elaboration at the amino groups that had complexed.

Zhao and co-workers received a patent describing preparation of 1-ethyl gentamicin C1a, a more potent gentamicin antibiotic than the naturally occurring gentamicin C1a, using the complexation concept. [24] First, a new mutant strain of *Micromonospora* was developed, which selectively produced only gentamicin component C1a, even though Gentamicin C1a could also have been produced by separating a mixture of components as noted above. Regioselective protection of gentamicin C1a by dropwise addition of a solution of acetic anhydride in tetrahydrofuran to a solution of the gentamicin C1a complexed with cobalt (II) acetate tetrahydrate in dimethylsulfoxide produced the 2',3,6'-tri-N-acetylgentamicin C1a in 80% yield (85% purity) after ion exchange chromatography via the methodology described above. Subsequent formation of a Schiff-base at C1 with acetaldehyde, followed by hydrogenation of the Schiff's base, provided regioselectively functionalized triacetylated 1-ethylgentamicin C1a. Basic deprotection followed by ion exchange chromatography provided good yields of 1-ethylgentamicin C1a [24].

Ghoshal also described complexation of gentamicin C1, here using two equivalents of the different divalent metal salt zinc acetate, in a nonaqueoous solvent (DMF). [25] The metal ions complexed with the same two pairs of polar groups previously noted, the C1 amino - C2'' hydroxyl pair as well as the C3'' amine - C4'' hydroxyl pair, rendering these functionalities unreactive and allowing selective protection at the remaining 2', 3, and 6' amino groups with di-tert-butyl dicarbonate. This permitted subsequent monofunctionalization at the reactive 3-amino group to occur when the uncomplexed product was subsequently reacted with electrophiles such as succinic anhydride and fluorescein isothiocyanate.

7

In order to develop an immunoassay, we required a single, monofunctionalized molecule of gentamicin. A single conjugate is preferable to a mixture of different conjugates, since a mixture of conjugates would be difficult to reproduce during repeated manufacturing.

Despite the previous observations on regioselective gentamicin functionalization, we believed that reaction conditions could be developed which would allow the gentamicin C1a isomer to be regioselectively monofunctionalized. Despite the fact that four of the amino groups in gentamicin C1a are primary, three of the amino groups are attached to secondary carbons, while only the 6'-amino group is attached to a carbon without alpha substitution. We thus theorized that this 6'-amino group would be more reactive due to steric constraints. This observation dovetailed nicely with our previously described results, in that fully protected gentamicin C1a was the first isomer to elute, providing the greatest number of unmixed fractions and making its separation from the other components straightforward.

For the monofunctionalization to be regioselective, mild reaction conditions and an electrophile with muted reactivity needed to be chosen. Since four of the amino groups were primary, more reactive electrophiles could conjugate at several of the amino groups, and provide complex mixtures from which the desired product would be difficult to separate. Of electrophiles with lowered reactivity, an active ester seemed to be the best choice. We preferred the pentafluorophenyl active ester as an acridinium active ester, because it offered muted reactivity as opposed to a succinimide or hydroxybenzotriazole ester and could provide a higher degree of steric congestion to its relatively larger planer aromatic ring. Low temperature conditions would encourage population of the lowest molecular conformation and provide the best chance for the reaction to be regioselective.

As expected, little selectivity for the amine group with no primary substitution was observed at ambient temperature. However, improved selectivity was observed at -55°C using a slow, dropwise addition of a solution of the acridinium pentafluorophenyl ester in dimethylformamide to a solution of the gentamicin C1a isomer in dimethylformamide in the presence of an amine base.

The reaction generated roughly 50% yields of the target acridinium conjugate after purification (Scheme 1, below). Attempts to improve the selectivity by lowering the temperature of the reaction provided mixtures that were difficult to stir, due to cooling of the solvent to nearly its freezing point, producing low selectivity for the desired amine group.

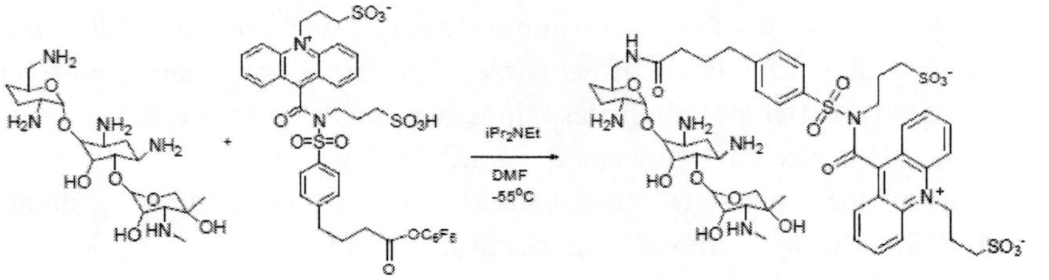

Scheme 1. Conjugation of pentafluorophenyl active ester with primary amine.

Confirmation of the identity of the major product as shown was obtained by electrospray mass spectrometry analysis of the purified conjugate, a tool that had previously been shown to have great utility in the degradation and identity of different gentamicin components This gentamicin derivative showed an $(M + H)^+$ at 1124.6 consistent with coupling of C1a to the acridinium label, and a strong fragment peak at 803.5 (calculated fragment mass 803.2) resulting from cleavage of the deoxystreptamine and garosamine residues, consistent with coupling to the purpurosamine ring (Figure 3). The proton NMR of the gentamicin C1a acridinium conjugate was also consistent with coupling to the 6'-amino group, showing a two proton doublet of doublets at d 4.23 (J = 7.3, J = 12.0 Hz), shifted from a two proton doublet of doublets at d 3.78 (J = 7.2 Hz, J = 12.0 Hz) observed for gentamicin C1a, consistent with conjugation to the primary amine on the purpurosamine ring that lacked alpha substitution.

Overall, the reproducible isolated three step yield of the regioselective conjugation after chromatography was 14-17% (27-33% based on the percent of gentamicin C1a present in lot of gentamicin complex used, based on the Certificate of Analysis), and the final tracer purity by HPLC was 96.7-99.3%.

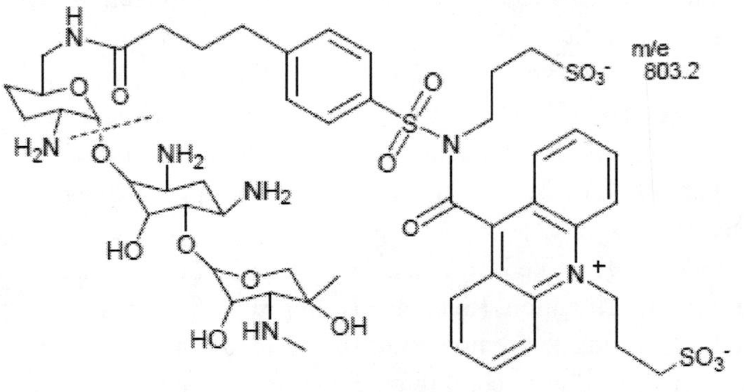

Figure 3. Fragmentation of gentamicin conjugate.

Since the conjugate was successfully used to develop an automated competitive immunoassay for gentamicin, [26] the antibody used was able to recognize and bind all three components of the complex in the presence of the gentamicin C1a conjugate.

In summary, the gentamicin complex is an aminoglycoside antibiotic consisting of three main components, each of which contains several different amino and hydroxyl groups. While some methods can successfully tolerate the use of the antibiotic complex without separation of its components, many authors have first separated the components to clarify their understanding of the utility of one component in a particular application. Other researchers have relied on the different environments which are present for the different amino groups, which allow for regioselective gentamicin protection and functionalization reactions. So long as new functionalized gentamicins continue to generate interest and provide useful improvements, the tools described above will permit virtually any novel gentamicin derivative that can be conceived to be synthesized.

REFERENCES

[1]   Prins, J.M.; Buller, H.R.; Kuijper, E.J.; Tange, R.A.; Speelman, P. *Lancet* 1993, *341*, 335–339.

[2]   Savic, M.; Ilic-Tomic, T.; MacMaster, R.; Vasilijevic, B.; Conn, G.L. *J. Bacteriology* 2008, *190*, 5855–5861.

[3]   Mugabe, C.; Halwani, M.; Azghani, A.O.; Lafrenie, R.M.; Omri, A. *Antimicrob. Agents Chemotherapy.* 2006, *50*, 2016–2022.

[4]   Lopez-Novoa, JM; Yaremi Quiros, Laura Vicente, Ana I Morales, Francisco J Lopez-Hernandez Kidney Int. 2011, 79(1), 33–45. (b) Sundin, D.P.; Sandoval, R.; Molitoris, B.A. *J. Am. Soc. Nephr.* 2001*, 12,* 114–123. (c) Sandoval, P.; *J. Am. Soc. Nephrol.* 1998, *7*, 167–174. (d) Tulkens, P. M. (1989). Nephrotoxicity of aminoglycoside antibiotics. *Toxicol. Lett* 46, 107–23.

[5]   Chu, J.; Zhang, S.; Zhuang, Y.; Chen, J.; Li, Y. *Process Biochemistry* (Oxford, UK) 2002, 38(5), 815–820.

[6]   Lauser, G., & Bergner, B. (1995) *Dtsch. Lebensm. Rundsch.*12, 390–396. (b) Stead, D., & Richards, R. (1997) *J. Chromatogr. B* 693, 415–421

[7]   Chen, Y.Q., Shang, Y.H., Li, X.M., Wu, X.P., & Xiao, X.L. *Food Chem.* 2008, *108*, 304–309.

[8]   Chen, Y.; Li, X.; He, L.; Tang, S.; Xiao, X.L. *J. AOAC Intl* 2012, *93*, 335–342.

[9]   Jin, Y.; Jin-Wook Jang, Mun-Han Lee and Chang-Hoon Han *Asian-Aust. J. Anim. Sci.* 2005, *18(10),* 1498–1504.

[10] Kadarugamuwa, J.L.; Clarke, AJ; Beveridge, T.J. *J. Bacteriology*, 1993, *175*, 5798–5805

[11] Schmid et al *Int. J. Physiol. Pathophysiol. Pharmacol.* 2011, *3*, 71.

[12] Karasawa, T.; Wang, O.; David, L.L.; and Steyger, P.S. *Toxicol. Sci.* 2011, 1–30.

[13] Claes, P.J.; Busson, R.; Vanderhaeghe, H. *J Chromatogr.* 1984, *298*, 445–447; (b) Wagman, P.; Marquez, J.A.; Weinstein, M.J. *J. Chromatogr.* 1968, *34*, 210–217; (c) Maehr, H.; Schaffner, C.P. *J. Chromatog*r. 1967, *30*, 572–578.

[14] Cooper, D.J.; Yudis, M.D.; Marigliano, M.; Traubei, T. *J. Chem. Soc., C.,* 1971, 2876–2879.

[15] Method essentially reproduced using HPLC in: Singh, P; Pirio, M.; Leung, D.K.; Tsay, Y. *Can. J. Chem.* 1984, *62*, 2471–2477.

[16] Grote, J. *US Patent Application* 2011, 0294994.

[17] Daniels, P.J.L.; Weinstein, J.; Nagabhushan, T.T. *J. Antibiotics* 1974, *27*, 889–893.

[18] Singh, P.H.; Pirio., M.; Leung, D.K.; Tsay, Y.-O. *Can. J. Chem.* 1984, *62*, 2471–2477.

[19] Wright, J.J. *US Patent* 4282350, 1981.

[20] Litovchick, A.; Evdokimov, A.R.; Lapidot, A. *FEB Letters* 1999, *445*, 73–79. (b) Litovchick, A.; Evdokimov, A.R.; Lapidot, *Biochemistry* 2000, 39, 2838–2852.

[21] Lapidot, A.; Litovchick, A. *Drug Disc. Res.* 2000, *50*, 502–515.

[22] Berchanski, A.; Lapidot, A. *Bioconjugate Chem.* 2008, *19,* 1896–1906.

[23] Nagabushan, T.L.; Cooper, AL.; et al. *J. Am. Chem. Soc.* 1978, *100*, 5253–5255.

[24] Zhao, M.; Fan, J.; Liu, J.; Hu, X.; Fan, M. *US Patent* 5,814,488, 1998.

[25] Ghoshal, M. *US Patent Application* 2003, 0060430.

[26] Grote, J.; Himmelsbach, R.; Johnson, D. *Tet. Lett* 2012, *53*, 6751–6754.

In: Gentamicin
Editor: Emilie Kruger

ISBN: 978-1-62808-841-0
© 2013 Nova Science Publishers, Inc.

Chapter 5

INDICATIONS AND ADVERSE EFFECTS OF GENTAMICIN

Lorena Giner-Bernal, Jaime Ruiz-Tovar, Antonio Arroyo, and Rafael Calpena
General University Hospital Elche, Alicante, Spain

ABSTRACT

Gentamicin is an antibiotic agent, belonging to the aminoglycosides group, which acts joining the ribosoma subunits 30S and 50S and blocking the translation of mRNA in the initial phase of protein synthesis, originating non-functional proteins in susceptible microorganisms [1]. Its bactericidal activity is concentration-dependent and is slightly influenced by the bacterial inoculum amount; the duration of the antibiotic effect ranges between 0.5-7 hours, depending on the concentration of antibiotic [2] and the exposure time to the drug [3].

Gentamicin acts inside the bacterial cell. This occurs in two stages by an active transport mechanism. In the first phase, the entrance into the cell depends on the transmembrane potential generated by aerobic metabolism. The second phase is favoured by the previous union of the aminoglycoside to the bacterial ribosome. Certain conditions that reduce the electrical potential of the membrane, such as anaerobic status or low pH of the medium, decrease the income of these compounds into the bacterial cytoplasm [4].

Once inside the cell, aminoglycosides join in an irreversible way the subunit 30S of the bacterial ribosome. This union interferes with the elongation of the peptide chain. They also cause incorrect translation of the genetic code, performing altered proteins. Some of these are membrane proteins and the result is the formation of channels that allow the entrance of more drug into the cell.

Specifically, gentamicin is active against gram-negative aerobic bacilli, including *Enterobacteriaceae* and non-fermenting microorganisms (excepting *Stenotrophomona maltophilia* and Burkholderia cepacia). It shows antibiotic action against Staphylococci [5] (*S. aureus* and *S. epidermidis*), including penicillinase-producing strains, but presents limited activity against *Streptococci*, lacking any activity against anaerobic bacteria and *Mycobacteria*. It is the most effective aminoglycoside against *Serratia* and *Brucella*, and presents the best synergic effect against *Streptococci, Enterococcus, Staphylococci* and *Listeria,* when combined with beta-lactam agents or vancomycin.

The cut-off point to determine the sensitivity of a microorganism to this antibiotic is with a CMI$\leq$4 mg/L. On the other hand, a bacteria can be considered resistant to gentamicin when presenting a CMI$\geq$16 mg/L. The maximal effect is obtained at concentrations of 6 - 10 mg/L with doses of 1.5 mg/kg iv or im. Gentamicin presents renal elimination at 90% and 10% with the bile [6].

INDICATIONS FOR GENTAMICIN ADMINISTRATION

Intra-Abdominal Infections

Gentamicin can be used in acute infections, such as appendicitis, cholecystitis, perforated ulcers, diverticulitis, pancreatitis, salpingitis, pelvic infections..., causing intra-abdominal abscess or peritonitis [7, 8, 9]. These pathologies tend to present polymicrobial infection, involving anaerobic and aerobic agents. Therefore, gentamicin should be associated with piperacilin-tazobactam, carbapenems or other drugs against anerobic microorganisms, such as metronidazole.

Skin and Soft Tissue Infections

Gentamicin can be used in combination with penicillin, clindamycin or carbapenems for infections involving mixed bacterial flora, as happens in necrotizing fasciitis or Fournier gangrene [10, 11].

Biliary Infections

Herein, the most important entities are cholangitis [12, 13] and cholecystitis. In both pathologies, the mostly involved bacteria are gram-negative bacilli, mainly *E.coli*. In these cases, it is common the association of gentamicin with a betalactam agent [14], because of their synergistic effect. Infections of biliary origin [15] are rising up, due to the increase of the interventionism in the biliary tree and the number of hepatobiliary surgeries. Around 80% of the infections are polymicrobian, representing a life-threatening condition because of its fesasability of producing bacteremia, (10% after cholecysitis and 50% after cholangitis).

The treatment of these conditions can include beta-lactams associated to gentamicin [16] or carbapenems.

Genitourinary Infections

In case of pyelonephritis or complicated urinary tract infections (UTI) or refractory ones and UTI associated with catheter, treatment might include the association of ampicillin and gentamicin, or just gentamicin in single dose.

Although *E. coli* remains the most common causative organism of UTI, when referring to agents causing nosocomial UTI, *Enterococcus spp., Pseudomonas spp.*, and fungi must be also taken into consideration.

Gentamicin is not indicated in first episodes of not complicated UTI, unless the microorganisms involved are resistant to antibiotics of less potential toxicity. In these cases, it is recommended to administrate a lower dose of gentamicin.

Bone Infections

As is the case of the osteomyelitis. Although aminoglycoside lose their effectiveness in acid media and do not show any action against anaerobes, gentamicin can be used in association with antibiotics against gram-positive pathogens, which are the most frequently causative agents of osteomyelitis (i.e. vancomycin).

Infections in Burned Patients

The burned surface is initially sterile, but from the second day onwards, there is a rapid bacterial colonization of the wound, mainly by gram-positive bacteria, which resisted the high temperatures of burn in the depth of sweat glands or hair follicles. After few days, there is also a colonization of the wound by gram-negative bacteria.

Most of the infections are monobacterian. Gram-positive bacteria do not usually trend to depth invasion, and generally do not exceed the fascias. However, gram-negative ones tend to affect underlying healthy tissues. The rapid proliferation of bacteria may induce ischemia and hemorrhage in the burned patient, increasing the depth of the infection. Consequently, secondary bacteremia and septic metastases might occur.

The most frequently isolated bacteria in the wound are *Staphylococci* (*S. aureus* in more than half of the cases, although the S. coagulase-negative are not uncommon) and gram-negative *Pseudomonas spp, Enterobacteriacea, Serratia spp,* etc.), and less frequently fungi (*Candida spp, Aspergillus*). Notwithstanding, flora is variable among different centres, according to the different periods or antibiotic strategies. We must also kept in mind, that oportunistic agents are unfrequent in burned wounds, but they can sometimes appear.

In the case of development of sepsis of cutaneous origin, it is necessary to begin a treatment, covering the most frequent agents (*Staphylococci* and gram-negative bacteria). Therefore, the empirical therapy[17] in sepsis of cutaneous origin should includes the administration of vancomycin associated with piperacillin-tazobactam, carbapenem, or fluoroquinolones in combination with aminoglycosides. When isolating the causant agents, antibiotic therapy must be revised according the antibiotic spectrum and their sensitivities. Surgical debridement is also an essential coadjuvant element in the treatment of sepsis of dermal origin.

Other Infections

Meningitis, septicemia, peritonitis, listeriosis, plague, pneumonia granuloma inguinale (*Klebsiella, Pseudomonas*), endocardytis or malignant external otitis, caused by *Pseudomonas* are infections amenable for treatment with gentamicin alone or in combination with other antibiotic drugs.

DOSING

The usual adult dose is 5 to 7 mg/kg/day in 1 or 2 doses, administered intramuscular or intravenously (diluted in normal saline with an infusion time of 30-60 minutes). In children the dose decreases to 3-7.5 mg/kg/day dose in 1 to 3 doses per day. Special attention is necessary in patients with renal failure, adjusting the dose depending on the levels of glomerular filtration. Moreover, gentamicin must be avoided during in pregnancy and in patients with liver function disorders.

INTERACTIONS [18, 19] AND ADVERSE EFFECTS

Gentamicin is incompatible with erythromycin, chloramphenicol, sulfadiazine, furosemide and sodium bicarbonate. Cisplatin decreases the elimination of gentamicin. It is a very nephrotoxic [20] drug, more even than tobramicin and amikacin, as well as ototoxic [21] affecting the vestibular portion of the State-acoustic nerve.

Generally, aminoglycosides have diverse adverse effects [22]

- Rarely produce hypersensitivity reactions, as well as phlebitis when administered intravenously.
- Exceptionally, they can cause a neuromuscular blockade (disruption of acetylcholine release in the presynaptic region by interference in the absorption of calcium), whose paralysis can be reversed with intravnous infusion of calcium gluconate. This risk is higher when the patients present basal hypocalcemia or hypomagnesemia, botulism, myasthenia gravis and when they are receiving treatment with calcium antagonists, colimicin, succinylcholine, or other drugs used in anesthesia for muscle relaxeation. Fast intravenous administration of high doses, especially in patients with renal failure, must be avoided, mainly to reduce the risk of appearance of these complitions.
- Gentamicin can produce cochlear lesions [23], as well as in the vestibular apparatus. The existence of a genetic predisposition in relation to the presence of mutations in the 12S rRNA has been described.
  - o Cochlear toxicity can be preceded by the emergence of tinnitus or feeling of fullness of the ear. The initial damage is manifested by

a high-frequency hearing loss [24] (the perception of the frequencies used in the hearing of the language is not changed). At this stage, the damages are usually reversible, but if the administration continues or the patient receives repeated cycles of treatment, hearing of spoken language can be also affected. In this phase, the damage is permanent or only partially reversible. Neomycin is the most toxic aminoglucoside drug to the cochlea, but differences in ototoxicity [25] between the rest of aminoglucosides are not significant.

o   Vestibular toxicity is characterized by the appearance of nausea, nystagmus, ataxia, vomiting and vertigo. It is most frequently observed when using streptomycin. Concomitant administration of furosemide or ethacrynic acid increases the risk of ototoxocity [26].

- Referring to nephrotoxicity [27], it might appear in 5-10% of patients, since this drugs tend to accumulate in lysosomes of the tubular epithelium. The first manifestations of their presence are the appearance of lysosomal enzymes, Beta-2-microglobulin and cylinders in the urine, phospholipidury, glycosury and urinary loss of potassium, magnesium and calcium. The lysosomes break and release enzymes causing cell necrosis and tubule-glomerular reflux, leading to local vasoconstriction and decreased glomerular filtration[28]. Clinically, acute renal failure might appear. Concomitant administration of NSAIDs may worsen renal failure. The progression of renal failure to the oliguric or anuric forms is very rare. The damage is reversible and usually improve within a few days, because, unlike the cochlear cells, the renal tubule can regenerate. The collection system of the aminoglycoside in the renal tubule[29] (by means of a protein known as anionic megolin) is saturable. The magnitude of the accumulation depends more on the time of persistence of the drug into the urine rather that to the urinary concentration. It has been also detected an increase in nephrotoxicity after concomitant administration of aminoglycosides and cephalosporins.

Table 1. Activity of gentamicin against diverse micro-organisms

SENSITIVE TO GENTAMICIN		RESISTANT TO GENTAMICIN*	
GRAM- NEGATIVES	*GRAM- POSITIVES*	*GRAM- NEGATIVES*	*GRAM- POSITIVES*
Escherichia coli	*Methicillin-sensitive*	*Acinetobacter baumannii*	*Streptococcus pneumoniae*
Proteus spp.	*Staphylococcus aureus*	*Burkholderia cepacea*	*Sreptococcus pyogenes*
Providencia spp.	*Coagulase negative*	*Stenotrophomonas maltophilia*	*Streptococcus spp*
Klebsiella spp.	*Staphylococcus methicillin sensitive*		*Enterococcus spp*
Enterobacter spp.			*Methicillin-resistant*
Serratia spp.**			*Staphylococcus aureus*
Citrobacter freundii			*Resistant coagulase negative*
Salmonella spp.			*Staphylococcus aureus*
Shigella spp.			
Yersinia pestis			
Pseudomonas aeruginosa			
Francisella tularensis			
Brucella abortus			

* Gentamicin does not show any activity against anaerobic microorganisms, *Rickettsia, Mycoplasma,* fungi or viruses.

** The gentamicin's CMI against *Serratia spp* is half than that of other aminoglycosides and it is considered the aminoglycoside of choice for infections caused by this bacterium.

REFERENCES

[1]   Abramowicz M, "Antimicrobial Prophylaxis in Surgery," Medical Letter on Drugs and Therapeutics, Handbook of Antimicrobial Therapy, 16th ed, New York, NY: *Medical Letter*, 2002

[2]   McLean AJ, IoannidesDemos LL, Li SC, et al. Bactericidal effect of gentamicin peak concentration provides a rationale for administration of bolus doses. *J Antimicrob Chemother* 1993; 32:301-305.

[3]   Begg EJ, Barclay ML, Duffull SB. A suggested approach to once-daily aminoglycoside dosing. *Br J Clin Pharmacol* 1995; 39:605-609.

[4]   Novelli A, Mazzei T, Fallani S, et al. In vitro postantibiotic effect and postantibiotic leukocyte enhancement of tobramycin. *J Chemother* 1995; 7:355-362.

[5]   Tam VH, Kabbara S, Vo G, et al. Comparative pharmacodynamics of gentamicin against Staphylococcus aureus and Pseudomonas aeruginosa. *Antimicrob Agents Chemother* 2006; 50:2626-2631.

[6]   Garrelts JC. Exploration of once-daily dosing of aminoglycosides through Bayesian simulation. Pharmacotherapy 1996; 16:286-294.

[7]   Such J, Runyon BA. Spontaneous bacterial peritonitis. Clin Infect Dis 1998; 27:669-676.

[8]   McHutchison JG, Runyon BA. Spontaneous bacterial peritonitis. In: Gastrointestinal and Hepatic Infections, Surawicz CM, Owen RL (Eds), WB Saunders, Philadelphia 1994; p.455.

[9]   Felisart J, Rimola A, Arroyo V, et al. Cefotaxime is more effective than is ampicillin-tobramycin in cirrhotics with severe infections. *Hepatology* 1985; 5:457-462.

[10]   Cosgrove SE, Vigliani GA, Fowler VG Jr, et al. Initial low-dose gentamicin for Staphylococcus aureus bacteremia and endocarditis is nephrotoxic. *Clin Infect Dis* 2009; 48:713-721.

[11]   Fortunov RM, Hulten KG, Hammerman WA, et al. Evaluation and treatment of community-acquired Staphylococcus aureus infections in term and late-preterm previously healthy neonates. *Pediatrics* 2007; 120:937-945.

[12]   Van den Hazel SJ, Speelman P, Tytgat GN, et al. Role of antibiotics in the treatment and prevention of acute and recurrent cholangitis. *Clin Infect Dis* 1994; 19:279-286.

[13]   Sinanan MN. Acute cholangitis. *Infect Dis Clin North Am* 1992; 6:571-599.

[14] Sung JJ, Lyon DJ, Suen R, et al. Intravenous ciprofloxacin as treatment for patients with acute suppurative cholangitis: a randomized, controlled clinical trial. J Antimicrob Chemother 1995; 35:855-864.

[15] Leung JW, Ling TK, Chan RC, et al. Antibiotics, biliary sepsis, and bile duct stones. *Gastrointest Endosc* 1994; 40:716-721.

[16] Gerecht WB, Henry NK, Hoffman WW, et al. Prospective randomized comparison of mezlocillin therapy alone with combined ampicillin and gentamicin therapy for patients with cholangitis. *Arch Intern Med* 1989; 149:1279-1284.

[17] Gilbert DN, Moellering RC, Eliopoulos GM, et al, eds, The Sanford Guide To Antimicrobial Therapy, 2006. 36th ed, Hyde Park, VT: Antimicrobial Therapy, Inc, 2006; 6-7.

[18] Dowell JA, Korth-Bradley J, Milisci M, et al, "Evaluating Possible Pharmacokinetic Interactions Between Tobramycin, Piperacillin, and a Combination of Piperacillin and Tazobactam in Patients With Various Degrees of Renal Impairment," *J Clin Pharmacol*, 2001; 41:979-86.

[19] Viollier AF, Standiford HC, Drusano GL, et al, "Comparative Pharmacokinetics and Serum Bactericidal Activity of Mezlocillin, Ticarcillin and Piperacillin, With and Without Gentamicin," *J Antimicrob Chemother*, 1985; 15:597-606.

[21] Smith CR and Lietman PS, "Effect of Furosemide on Aminoglycoside-Induced Nephrotoxicity and Auditory Toxicity in Humans," *Antimicrob Agents Chemother*, 1983; 23:133-7.

[22] Matz GJ, "Aminoglycoside Ototoxicity," *Am J Otolaryngol*, 1986; 7:117-9.

[23] O'Brien RK and Sparling TG, "Gentamicin and Fludarabine Ototoxicity," *Ann Pharmacother*, 1995; 29(2):200-1.

[24] Hatala R, Dinh T, Cook DJ. Once-daily aminoglycoside dosing in immunocompetent adults: a meta-analysis. *Ann Intern Med* 1996; 124:717-725.

[25] Contopoulos-Ioannidis DG, Giotis ND, Baliatsa DV, Ioannidis JP. Extended-interval aminoglycoside administration for children: a meta-analysis. *Pediatrics* 2004; 114:e111.

[26] Rybak MJ, Abate BJ, Kang SL, et al. Prospective evaluation of the effect of an aminoglycoside dosing regimen on rates of observed nephrotoxicity and ototoxicity. *Antimicrob Agents Chemother* 1999; 43:1549-1555.

[27] Mulheran M, Hyman-Taylor P, Tan KH, et al. Absence of cochleotoxicity measured by standard and high-frequency pure tone

audiometry in a trial of once- versus three-times-daily tobramycin in cystic fibrosis patients. *Antimicrob Agents Chemother* 2006; 50:2293-2299.

[28] Halstenson CE, Wong MO, Herman CS, et al, "Effect of Concomitant Administration of Piperacillin on the Dispositions on Isepamicin and Gentamicin in Patients With End-Stage Renal Disease," *Antimicrob Agents Chemother*, 1992. 36:1832-36.

[29] Heintz BH, Matzke GR, Dager WE, "Antimicrobial Dosing Concepts and Recommendations for Critically Ill Adult Patients Receiving Continuous Renal Replacement Therapy or Intermittent Hemodialysis," *Pharmacotherapy*, 2009. 29:562-77.

INDEX

D

E

F

T